EAT

CHEW

LIVE

What Medical Professionals Say about *Eat, Chew, Live*

"A fascinating inquisition into the metabolic machinery of the human body with common sense advice on diabetes prevention."

—**Sumit Bhagra, MD, FACE, Endocrinologist,
Mayo Clinic Health System**

"As a physician and a prediabetic, my fascination with reading this book was personal. Books on diabetic solutions are many, but EAT CHEW LIVE is unique in that it does not prescribe any diets, provide recipes, or sell products. It suggests that the way we eat is the most effective tool to control our diabetes. I tried his suggested methods, including eliminating consumption of complex carbohydrates and taking time to chew. I was able to lose five pounds and lower my fasting blood sugar within a seven-week period. I did not use any anti-diabetic medications during this time.

I fully endorse this book for anyone who cares about his or her health and wants to live a full life. While the politics of pharmaceutical management of diabetes mellitus and the medical establishment may resist these ideas, I foresee a paradigm shift in the understanding of the cause of diabetes and how it can be prevented, reversed, or controlled using Dr. Poothullil's methods. Dr. Poothullil's decades of painstaking research and his revolutionary ideas are worth paying close attention to."

—**A. E. Daniel, MD, DPM, MRC Psych, Distinguished Life Fellow of the
American Psychiatric Association, Adjunct Professor of Psychiatry,
University of Missouri School of Medicine**

"There has been a dramatic increase in the incidence of Type 2 diabetes in the United States and worldwide over the last few decades, coincident with the obesity epidemic. One-third of the U.S. population, both children and adults, is either overweight or obese. Unless something changes, the U.S. Centers for Disease Control and Prevention (CDC) predicts that one-third of babies born in the year 2000 will develop diabetes.

In his book, Dr. Poothullil challenges the concept of "insulin resistance," pointing out that there is no clear scientific explanation for the mechanism of cell resistance to the effect of insulin. Dr. Poothullil instead presents a different, novel hypothesis to explain abnormally elevated blood sugar levels. His provocative ideas will challenge physicians who care for patients with diabetes to rethink the paradigm of insulin resistance and current modes of treatment for patients with Type 2 diabetes."

—Stephen H. LaFranchi, M.D., Professor, Pediatric Endocrinology,
Oregon Health Sciences University

"This book is very readable. The science is understandable and backed up with analogies, such as how cells use more than one kind of fuel similar to a hybrid car. Dr. Poothullil's presents a provocative, new hypothesis on Type 2 diabetes, and its care and prevention. After reading Chapter 22, "Enemy #1—Our Grain-Based Culture," I believe nobody will be able to look at cereal, rice, and bread again without remembering it all turns into sugar inside the body."

—Janet Meirelles, BSN, RN, Certified Diabetes Educator,
author of *Diabetes Is Not a Piece of Cake*

JOHN M. POOTHULLIL, MD, FRCP

EAT

CHEW

LIVE

4 Revolutionary Ideas to
Prevent Diabetes, Lose Weight
and Enjoy Food

Editorial Direction and Editing: Rick Benzel
Copyeditor: Marian Pierce
Art Direction and Cover Design: Susan Shankin & Associates
Interior Design: Tanya Maiboroda
Cover Illustration and Special Insert Illustrations: Tim Kummerow
Text Illustrations: CristianVoicu
Author Photo: Pete Perry
Published by Over And Above Press
Over And Above Creative Group, Los Angeles, CA
www.overandabovecreative.com

First edition

Library of Congress Control Number: 2015901721

ISBN: 978-0-9907924-0-6

Visit our website and blog for updates and to submit your questions:
www.eatchewlive.com
questions@eatchewlive.com

Distributed by SCB Distributors

1 in 3 adults in the U.S. over age 20 is prediabetic,
meaning he or she has high blood sugar.
9 out of 10 of them do not know they have it.
1 to 3 will develop diabetes within 5 years.

This book will tell you how to avoid developing high blood sugar.

■

1 in 11 adults in the U.S. over age 20 has diabetes.
1 in 4 do not know they have it.

This book will tell you how to reverse your diabetes.

Dedicated to the memory of

Jerry Dolovich MD (1997),

McMaster University,

Hamilton, Ontario, Canada,

who encouraged me to think beyond the obvious.

CONTENTS

PART 3

Reconnecting with Your Authentic Weight

PART 4

Eat What You Enjoy & Enjoy What You Eat

"Let food be your medicine."

CREDITED TO HIPPOCRATES

I wrote *Eat, Chew, Live* for people who are concerned about their eating habits, are gaining weight or are already obese, or who have high blood sugar or Type 2 diabetes. This is a growing segment of the world's population because obesity and diabetes are becoming two of the top health problems in the US as well as throughout the developed world. I invite you to read this book if:

- you are gaining weight or have become obese and cannot control your eating habits,
- your doctor has asked you to change your eating habits and lifestyle,
- you believe you are at risk for getting diabetes because it is in your family,
- your doctor has detected that you have a higher than normal blood sugar level,
- you have been diagnosed with "prediabetes" and are taking medication to control it,
- your doctor told you that you have prediabetes, but you don't want to take medication to control it,
- you have a family member or friend who has a higher blood sugar than normal or who has been diagnosed with prediabetes and you want to help them learn how to prevent diabetes,
- you are a counselor working for a public or private agency that counsels people about prediabetes and diabetes,
- you are a medical doctor who is willing to learn a more useful and accurate explanation for the cause of prediabetes and diabetes in your patients and the most effective ways to reverse it.

If you are currently a diabetic, the recommendations in this book can also help your blood sugar levels eventually return to normal, effectively "reversing" your diabetes and possibly allowing you to stop taking medication. If you were recently diagnosed with "full-blown" diabetes, there may still be time to lower your high blood sugar condition by following the advice in this book.[1]

Four Revolutionary Ideas

Not long after I began practicing medicine, I became interested in understanding the causes of and interconnections between hunger, satiation, and weight gain. My interest turned into a passion and a multi-decade personal study and research project that led me to read many medical journal articles, medical textbooks, and other scholarly works in biology, biochemistry, physiology, endocrinology, and cellular metabolic functions. This eventually guided me to investigate the theory of insulin resistance as it relates to diabetes. Recognizing that this theory made no sense, I spent a few years rethinking the biology behind high blood sugar and I began developing the ideas in this book.

Eat, Chew, Live presents my four revolutionary ideas that can help you change your relationship to food, learn to stop overeating, lose weight, and prevent diabetes. My recommendations are based on a scientific approach, summarized by these four concepts:

- Overeating causes your body's muscle cells to switch from using glucose for cellular energy to using fatty acids, leaving the glucose in your bloodstream. This is the cause of diabetes rather than the widely accepted theory of insulin resistance.
- Our brain is set up to select, regulate, and track our consumption and usage of nutrients to supply our body's cells; you can teach yourself to listen to your brain to avoid overeating.
- Becoming aware of your "authentic weight" is the key to regaining the motivation to eat properly and avoid the foods that cause weight gain and high blood sugar.

---

[1] Reversing diabetes will not repair any damage the disease may have already caused, such as damage to your nerves (diabetic neuropathy), eye problems, kidney problems, or heart conditions.

- Relearning to eat with the same mindful consciousness you had as a child will enable you to respect your body's nutritional needs and not overwhelm it with glucose and fat.

You will find my ideas and recommendations to be quite different from anything else you have ever read or heard. Although I advocate for losing weight, not eating carbohydrates, and better eating habits, I present these recommendations from a very different angle than other doctors, nutritionists, and weight loss advisors. In my decades of practicing medicine as an allergist and pediatrician, I have spent countless hours thinking about obesity, diabetes, and the relationship between eating and nutrition. After years of thought and research, I have developed what I believe is a more scientifically accurate explanation than insulin resistance for why people gain weight and develop Type 2 diabetes. My four revolutionary ideas also reflect a completely new approach to understanding how to lose weight and keep it off, while avoiding diabetes and learning how to eat healthy food in a "mindful" way.

In fact, just as this book was in its final stages of publishing, a new study confirmed that four highly popular diets do not work *on a long-term basis* to lose weight and eliminate body fat, both of which are the keys to preventing high blood sugar and the onset of diabetes.[2] People often say they know this, but they still spend billions of dollars on diet programs and diet foods. Of course, diets—the restriction of energy intake—can result in weight loss (the best example is starving), but in order to prevent regaining the lost weight, you have to correct the way you were consuming energy-containing foods before the weight gain started in the first place; otherwise the cycle of weight gain and diet simply repeats itself.

In order to practice the "correct" way of eating—a way that allows your body to match the intake of energy-containing foods to what it needs—you have to understand the normal way of eating, and more importantly, how YOU deviated from that. In short, you have to relearn *HOW to eat* because that determines how much you eat and how much you weigh. To stop gaining

---

[2] Eisenberg MJ. et.al., *Long-term benefits of popular diets are less than evident,* American Heart Association Rapid Access Journal Report November 11, 2014 Categories: Heart News.

weight and avoid diabetes, you have to relearn how to savor the food in your mouth, and this is what I will teach you.

Developing Diabetes is a Serious Risk

Why should you be concerned about diabetes? The answer is, you may already be among the 1 in 3 adults in the US who has prediabetes but do not know it. Even if you are thin or have no family history of diabetes, you could have high blood sugar and be on your way to becoming diabetic. If you are an adult in your 30s, 40s, or 50s who has been gaining weight for years, you are possibly at risk for developing high blood sugar or diabetes within several more years.

It is frightening that the incidence of Type 2 diabetes is skyrocketing in the US and elsewhere in the world. It is fast becoming one of the most serious health risks for millions of people. Here are the most recent estimates from the Centers for Disease Control and Prevention (published in 2014 and based on data from 2012) that are worth keeping in mind as you read this book:[3]

- 86 million Americans older than age 20 have prediabetes—that's roughly 1 in 3 adults in the US aged 20 years or older. Nearly 93% of these people do not even know they have it.
- 29 million American adults have Type 2 diabetes. Almost 30% of this number are unaware they have it.
- Of the 29 million with diabetes, about 11 million are over age 65. That's 1 in 4 seniors with diabetes.
- Diabetes is the 7th leading cause of death in the US. About 300,000 people die each year with diabetes listed as the primary or a contributing cause of death.

Diabetes is a serious medical condition. Below are some of the health problems that uncontrolled Type 2 diabetes causes:

---

[3] http://www.cdc.gov/diabetes/pubs/statsreport14/national-diabetes-report-web.pdf and http://www.cdc.gov/images/campaigns/nccdphp/diabetes-infographic.jpg

- *Damage to body cells, leading to diabetic neuropathy.* When blood glucose levels stay consistently high, glucose can attach to proteins of cells such as nerve cells, interfering with their function.
- *Atherosclerosis, leading to heart attack, stroke, or the need to amputate limbs.* Diabetes can lead to hardening of the arteries that reduces blood flow to cells in the heart, brain, or limbs.
- *Potential organ failure, leading to blindness or the need for dialysis due to kidney failure.* Uncontrolled glucose levels in the blood damage the small blood vessels in the eyes and kidneys.
- *Impotence in men, leading to erectile dysfunction.* Diabetes can reduce blood flow to the penis and make it difficult to have an erection.
- *Diabetic coma.* A person with Type 2 diabetes who becomes severely dehydrated and is unable to drink enough fluids to make up for the fluid losses can go into a diabetic coma.

Decades ago, Type 2 diabetes was called "adult onset" because the typical age of onset was over 60 years. Today, people in their 30s or 40s get diabetes. Some are diagnosed as early as their 20s and younger. Once you get high blood sugar, it can persist throughout your lifetime unless you do something to control it. But you can prevent diabetes in a completely natural way if you follow the concepts and advice in this book.

Eat, Chew, Live will help you gain a radical new understanding of your relationship with food. I will be teaching you about your body and brain, and helping you develop a new awareness of food and how you eat it. This knowledge will keep you healthy and diabetes-free. This book does not prescribe any special diet or ask you to buy any products. All I ask of you is to Eat, Chew, and Live.

PART 1

A Revolutionary

New Theory

about the

Cause of Diabetes

He who distinguishes the true savor of
his food can never be a glutton.

—HENRY DAVID THOREAU

CHAPTER 1

The Disease You Never Expect to Get!

Return to the days when you were 14 years old—a happy, growing teenager. The thought that you'll develop health problems in the future never crosses your mind. You spend the afternoon at school gym class playing baseball, race around with some friends after school and then run to catch the bus. By the time you arrive home, you're ravenous. You grab some slices of bread and make a peanut butter and jelly sandwich. After scarfing it down with a glass of milk, you're still hungry, so you microwave a slice of leftover pizza. You're an active teen so you're still not satisfied, and now you munch an apple. You would keep eating but remember that your mom is making her special spaghetti dinner and decide to leave room for it.

Why do you need all this food when you are 14? At that age, your body craves nutrients to power your muscles, your brain cells, and the cells of all your organs. What happens to all the food you ate? The acid in your stomach and contractions of the stomach muscle break your "snack" down into particles that enter your small intestine, where the particles are digested by enzymes into the nutrients your body needs.

Anything you ate that contained complex carbohydrates, such as the bread and pizza dough, break down in the small intestine first to *maltose*, and then to the most basic form of carbohydrate, called *glucose*. Dairy products like milk and cheese have a form of sugar called *lactose*, and this, too, may eventually be changed into glucose. Fruits contain a natural sugar, *sucrose*, which may also be broken down into glucose. The rest of the foods you eat break down into fatty acids, amino acids, cholesterol, minerals, vitamins, and many other micronutrients that the cells of your body need to function.[1]

All the absorbed nutrients enter the general blood circulation for a journey to their destinations—the millions of cells in your body. As nutrient absorption into your bloodstream continues, all the carbohydrates that have ultimately broken down into glucose cause your 'blood sugar' level to climb.

But you are young and spent the afternoon expending energy. Now your body needs more. Glucose is the primary fuel used to power our brain cells and red blood cells. Our muscles can use either glucose or the fatty acids derived from various foods such as meats, fish, nuts, milk and butter for energy. Your skeletal muscles are like a hybrid car that can use electricity or gasoline to run the engine. If glucose is present, they will use that first, but if it is not present, the body will start to convert the fat stored in your fat cells into fatty acids that your cells can use for energy.

The good news is that your youthful teenage body begins to use much of the glucose from your snack almost immediately. Because your muscle cells have been activated from the exercise, glucose easily enters them (figure 1). Ordinarily, *insulin*, the hormone produced in the pancreas, is necessary to "ease" the way for glucose to enter your cells. However, cells do not need help from insulin to let glucose in when they are active. In fact, the brain, liver, and activated muscle cells do not need the assistance of insulin to let glucose in.

---

[1] An interesting side note: If our scenario were taking place in a part of the world that has little access to complex carbohydrates such as wheat, corn, and other grains and fresh fruits, your teenage liver is likely to have adapted over generations of time to produce glucose using protein rather than carbohydrates. For example, people living in the sub-arctic regions often survive on a diet consisting of mostly animal fat and protein rather than grains, rice, potatoes, and fruit. Their genetic code has reprogrammed their liver to use amino acids, the products of protein breakdown, to produce glucose. The liver's capability of producing glucose from protein is actually important for survival in parts of the world where climate conditions prevent the cultivation of plants that produce complex carbohydrates. This population has bigger livers with a larger capacity for converting protein to glucose.

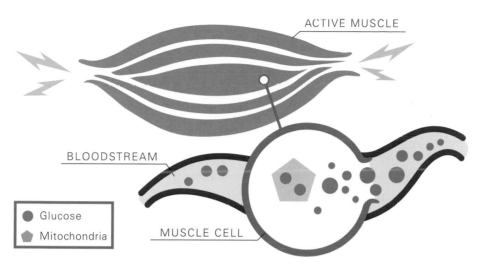

Figure 1. Active muscle cells can let glucose in without the presence of insulin. Muscles use glucose as fuel for their energy.

Glucose Absorption When Your Body is Cooled Down

Now jump to dinner time that evening. At 7:00 pm, you join your family to eat your mom's wonderful spaghetti and sauce, with homemade garlic bread. Your sister is vegetarian, but you are not, so you also consume five turkey meatballs. For dessert, you eat a yummy éclair filled with custard and 30 minutes later gobble down a banana.

Within a half-hour after finishing dinner, your stomach has begun transferring the food to your small intestine, which breaks it down further into smaller molecules. The spaghetti and bread are starches (carbohydrates) that get broken down, as explained earlier, into glucose. Portions of the tomato sauce break down into vitamins and minerals but other portions into glucose. The cream filling in the éclair and the banana you ate also contribute glucose. The protein part of the turkey meatballs is broken down into amino acids. The fat part contributes fatty acids and cholesterol. All these elements enter your bloodstream. All nutrients except for fat then flow to the liver where they are cleansed, and continue on their journey to the heart which pumps them throughout the body. Fat molecules enter the bloodstream directly, without having to go through the liver first (figure 2).

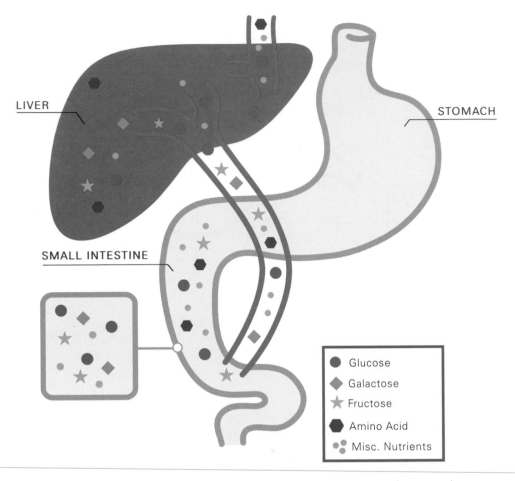

Figure 2. In digestion, food in the intestine is broken down into its component elements and nutrients. All nutrients except for fat then flow to the liver where they are cleansed, and continue on their journey to the heart which pumps them throughout the body. Fat molecules enter the bloodstream directly, without having to go through the liver first.

But what happens after dinner is different than after eating your afternoon snack. Your muscles have cooled down and become more inactive. The glucose from dinner is flooding your bloodstream, but this time it is not absorbed immediately into your muscles. As a result, your body sends a signal to the pancreas to begin producing and releasing insulin, a hormone whose molecules are like doormen standing outside the muscle cells, telling them to let the glucose in.

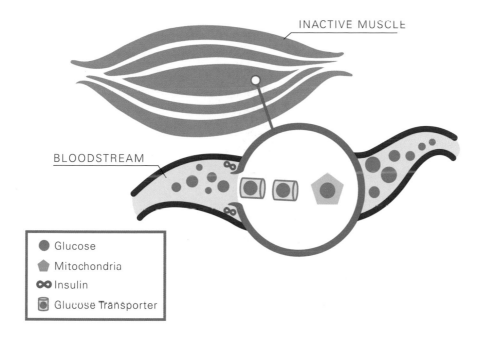

INACTIVE MUSCLE

BLOODSTREAM

- ● Glucose
- ⬠ Mitochondria
- ∞ Insulin
- ▣ Glucose Transporter

Figure 3. Insulin molecules attach to receptors on the cell wall, attracting transport modules within to capture glucose molecules outside the cell wall and guide them in to the cell.

When cells detect the presence of insulin outside their wall, they release "transport modules" from a holding area inside the cell. These help cut a "channel" in the cell wall for the glucose molecules to enter (figure 3).

The glucose molecules are then guided to a site in the cell called the mitochondria where they are used to produce ATP, which stands for *adenosine triphosphate.* ATP is the chemical your cells use to power their functions. Each cell prefers to use glucose to produce ATP, but as mentioned, they can also use fatty acids in the bloodstream to produce it (figure 4).[2]

Millions of molecules of ATP float around in each cell, ready to unload energy. Once made, most ATP molecules are used up within about two minutes, but some remain unused, ready to be activated whenever your body needs energy. Like the batteries of a flashlight, ATP is available to power your body when it needs it.

---

[2] Guyton and Hall, *Medical Physiology*, Twelfth Edition, 2011, Saunders Elsevier.

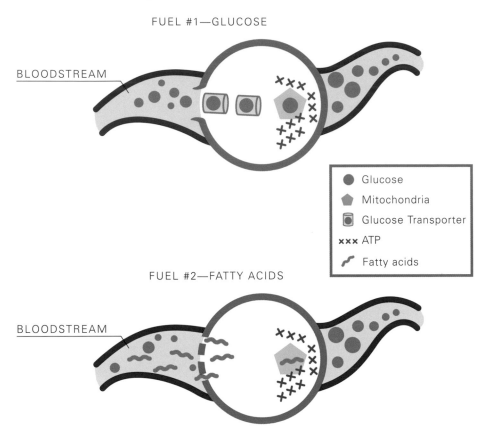

FUEL #1—GLUCOSE

BLOODSTREAM

Glucose
Mitochondria
Glucose Transporter
ATP
Fatty acids

FUEL #2—FATTY ACIDS

BLOODSTREAM

Figure 4. Your cells are like a hybrid car. They can use either glucose or fatty acids to produce ATP, the energy that powers cell functions.

Insulin is therefore a critical agent in metabolizing glucose for ATP when your muscles are inactive. In fact, the rate of glucose transport into most cells increases up to ten times the normal rate when insulin is present outside the cell wall than when insulin is not present.

What Happens to Glucose You Don't Burn?

The liver converts some glucose into glycogen and keeps it as the stored form of glucose. Insulin promotes this process. Glycogen is similar in configuration to that of starch from complex carbohydrates. Between meals, when your body needs more energy than the ATP already stored in the cells, the liver breaks glycogen back down again into glucose and ships it out on a fairly regular basis in an effort to maintain a constant blood sugar level. Insulin also plays a role in this process by preventing the liver from breaking down glycogen when there is already sufficient glucose in your bloodstream.

The body has another backup system for energy storage. Some of the excess glucose in your liver is converted to fatty acids. The liver uses these fatty acids, along with the other fatty acids from the food you eat, to manufacture *triglycerides*. Insulin promotes this process too. The liver sends the triglycerides to the fat storage cells in your tummy, thighs, buttocks and many other places of the body, where it waits to be used when your glucose levels decrease (figure 5).

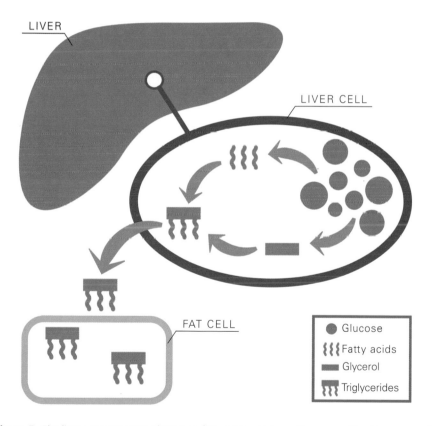

Figure 5. The liver converts some glucose to fatty acids which are then recombined in groups of three with a glycerol molecule to form triglyceride. The triglycerides are sent to your fat cells for storage.

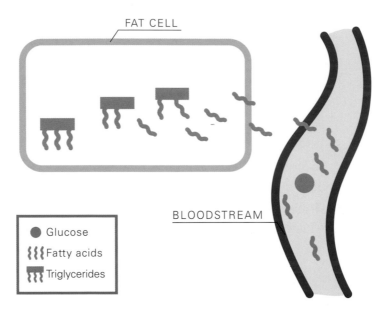

FAT CELL

BLOODSTREAM

- ● Glucose
- ⦃⦃⦃ Fatty acids
- ⦙⦙⦙ Triglycerides

Figure 6. Between meals or when exercising, if the body needs energy, triglycerides in your fat cells are broken down into fatty acids, which exit the cell and travel through the bloodstream to muscle cells that convert them to energy.

When your body needs more energy and your blood sugar drops below its required level, another hormone from the pancreas called *glucagon* prompts the liver to release glucose. In addition, glucagon facilitates reconversion of the triglycerides stored in your fat cells back into fatty acids for the muscles to burn in place of glucose (figure 6). The body also releases adrenaline to augment this process.

To summarize our teenager scenario, both the snack you ate in the afternoon and the dinner you had in the evening replenished your body with glucose that it used to nourish your brain cells, help your red blood cells stay oxygenated and healthy, and power your muscles. The difference between the two meals is that when you ate the snack, your muscles were still activated from exercising, whereas after dinner, your muscles had become inactive and your body needed insulin from your pancreas to help escort glucose into your muscle cells. Since you are a healthy teenager, utilizing the abundant glucose quickly from your bloodstream and having your pancreas produce insulin that ensures the glucose gets into your cells prevented you from developing too high a level of blood sugar.

You may have picked up this book because you were thinking about weight gain, high blood sugar, prediabetes or diabetes. Chances are that when you were a teenager, you never imagined you might become diabetic at some point in your life.

KEY POINTS

- All carbohydrates you eat are ultimately broken down in the small intestine and can be converted into glucose.

- Your cells can burn glucose or fatty acids to make ATP, the chemical that powers your cells.

- Inactive muscle cells need the presence of insulin, produced in the pancreas, to enable transport molecules in the cells to cut a channel for glucose to enter.

EAT CHEW LIVE was a real eye-opener for me. Its insights on the real causes of Type 2 diabetes are fascinating and challenge conventional thinking. Most importantly, I found it convincing. This made it easier for me to follow Dr. Poothullil's advice. I am enjoying food a lot more, while needing to eat a lot less. I have been successful for three years now in keeping my weight off and maintaining my blood sugar well below the threshold for prediabetes.

Jacob, Prediabetic, Oregon

CHAPTER 2

Three Scenarios of Diabetics

Let's jump ahead and meet three people who were active teenagers themselves but who developed prediabetes or diabetes as adults. Perhaps one of these teens will remind you of yourself. My goal in telling you these stories is to help you become aware that maintaining the same eating habits you had an as active teen can cause prediabetes or diabetes.

Steve

Steve is 62 years old. For most of his early adult life, he stayed within his weight/height ratio—5'9" and 160 pounds. By the time he was 35, Steve had two children and his life became much busier both at work and at home. Meals became a very important part of his day. He could finally relax and enjoy his wife and two young daughters. Both Steve and his wife loved to cook sumptuous meals. They also loved to entertain on the weekends, and often invited guests over for dinner.

By the time he was 45, Steve weighed 170, a 10 pound gain over 10 years. He played softball on weekends, but that was his only exercise. He loved eating well, especially thick sandwiches on crusty bread for lunch and dinners of pasta and sausages, roast beef and potatoes and chicken stew on rice. He often craved Chinese and Thai food with noodles, and pizza with the works. The years began ticking off and Steve's daughters grew up and started college. At 55, Steve weighed 180 pounds, with an extended belly like many men his age. He biked and went for occasional walks, but did not lose weight because he continued overeating.

At age 58, Steve went to his doctor for a physical and the doctor took his blood. A week later, the doctor's office called and asked him to come in. The doctor broke the news that he was prediabetic. Steve's mother and her two sisters all had Type 2 diabetes, but Steve never imagined that his own blood sugar would climb so high.

Here's how his doctor could tell Steve was prediabetic. When blood sugar levels are high, the glucose molecules attach to the hemoglobin in red blood cells in a process called *glycation*. The longer a person has high blood glucose levels, the higher the level of glycated hemoglobin. This can be measured in a test called the "A1C." Steve's doctor explained that anyone who has an A1C level between 5.7 and 6.4% is considered prediabetic, at risk for becoming a Type 2 diabetic. A full diabetic is someone whose A1C is over 6.5. Steve's A1C was at 6.4.

Steve was shocked. His doctor explained that it would be necessary for Steve to go on medication to bring his blood sugar under control. If Steve could bring the A1C back down, he could reverse his prediabetic condition and prevent himself from getting diabetes. But if his A1C climbed above 6.5 and remained there for a long time, it would be difficult to prevent complications such as dehydration, blood vessel damage to the eyes, nerve damage in the feet, inefficient filtration through the kidneys, and elevation of blood pressure. These complications from diabetes are hard to detect in the early stages because the symptoms usually don't appear until the damage has become serious.

Steve never understood why he suddenly became prediabetic. He had heard about the body's need for insulin to control blood sugar, but was unaware of the biological mechanisms involved. His doctor did not explain whether Steve had insulin resistance or a shortfall of insulin production in his pancreas. And, like most patients, Steve never asked. The doctor put Steve on a drug that stimulated his pancreas to produce more insulin. He told Steve to eat smaller portions and watch his intake of sweets, fruits, and carbohydrates. He also had Steve talk with a nutritionist for 30 minutes.

Steve is now 63 and has been taking the same prescription drug since his diagnosis. He has cut his weight down to 173, but the doctor has Steve come in for a blood test every 90 days. Steve still has difficulty eating smaller portions and not overeating. He has no idea whether he must take his medication forever, increase its dosage, or eventually encounter diabetic complications. He will hopefully read this book and begin to recognize that he can reverse his condition if he takes control.

Sam

Sam was a healthy, active teenager who played tennis and ran on the school's track team. But after developing a taste for beer and partying in college, he was 20 pounds overweight by the time he graduated. Sam then worked as an accountant in a major firm in his city, and over the years, he rose in the ranks to become a vice-president.

Sam loved to eat and his position in the company allowed him to take clients out frequently. His usual choice was an appetizer, followed by a steak or prime rib, baked potato or French fries, a vegetable, and chocolate cake or apple pie. By the time he was 40, Sam weighed 190 and his friends began politely calling him "portly." In another five years, he weighed 220.

At age 48, Sam was diagnosed as a diabetic. He never imagined he'd develop this condition despite decades of putting on weight and a family history of diabetes—his older sister had the disease. He took oral medication for several years, but his blood sugar continued to climb. Finally, his doctor decided that Sam's pancreas could no longer produce enough insulin and put Sam on three injections of insulin daily to supplement what his pancreas could produce. Sam checked his blood sugar twice daily by pricking his finger and using a meter to assess his blood sugar. His doctor allowed him to adjust his insulin dosage based on the reading. He was proud to keep his A1C below 7, but in effect he was still diabetic.

Today Sam is 70 and retired. But he is not living the life he expected in his retirement years. The doctor says his kidneys are beginning to fail because of cell damage from the diabetes. As I write this, Sam is trying to decide on stomach surgery to lose weight as his final stand before accepting the consequences of complete kidney failure.

Lisa

Lisa played volleyball in high school and was on the cheerleading team. She was fit and active, an attractive girl at 5′5″ and 110 pounds. Her mom was on the heavy side but her dad was lean and Lisa seemed to have inherited her father's physique.

Lisa married young and had a baby when she was 22. After she got pregnant, she was shocked to learn she had developed gestational diabetes and had high blood sugar, just like a diabetic. Gestational diabetes is a condition that some pregnant women get. Her doctor put her on medication to control her blood sugar and told her to watch her diet. After delivery, her blood sugar returned to normal and Lisa no longer had to take the medication.

When Lisa's daughter was 10, Lisa went back to work at an insurance company. She often ate lunch at her desk, but on occasion went out for pizza or a burger with her colleagues. In the evenings, she made a good meal for her daughter and husband. As she cooked, she usually drank a glass or two of wine—a little treat she offered herself after a hard day in the office. Lisa loved the outdoors, so on weekends she'd go biking or take her daughter swimming at the local YMCA. However, over the years, Lisa stopped exercising, claiming a lack of free time on weekends. She began to put on a few pounds. When she was 35 she weighed 120, but that was still within the "normal" range for her age and height.

Seven years later, Lisa was told that she was prediabetic. A specialist said it had nothing to do with her prior bout of gestational diabetes, nor was it a case of weight gain, since at 130 pounds Lisa was still within the normal range for her age. The doctors said that Lisa had simply developed "insulin resistance," when the cells of her body do not recognize the presence of insulin outside their cell walls, allowing glucose to accumulate in the blood and raise her blood sugar level. The doctor prescribed a medication to help Lisa's body's cells reduce their resistance to insulin, and asked her to measure her blood sugar two hours after meals on a regular basis.

At age 47, Lisa continued taking the medications, but a promotion led her to spend more hours in the office. She had also gained weight and believed the medication had caused it. She was frightened when her doctor told her that she was at "high risk" for developing blockage of the blood vessels to the heart, brain, and legs because of steadily increasing levels of fat in her blood vessels.

Jump ahead 20 years. Lisa is now 67. The complications of her diabetes have worsened over the decades. Despite taking both oral medication and insulin shots, she developed severe blood vessel blockage in her right leg, causing significant restriction of blood flow throughout her lower leg. Nothing the doctors tried to save her leg worked, and a year ago, they had to amputate it below the knee.

■

As teenagers, Steve, Sam and Lisa never imagined they would spend their adult lives struggling to control their diabetes. What about you? My goal in writing this book is to give you the tools to enjoy living free of the fear of developing diabetes or, if you already have diabetes, to find out how you can become healthy.

KEY POINT

■ Many people grow into adulthood not taking control of their weight or their food intake. The end result is they become overweight, obese, prediabetic or diabetic.

> ## "With an excess of fat diabetes begins, and from an excess of fat diabetics die."
> **Elliot P. Joslin, MD, Founder Joslin Diabetes Center** [1]

Now that you know that diabetes can be a serious condition, let's take a look at the accepted theory of diabetes called "insulin resistance." As explained, the pancreas releases insulin in response to elevation of the glucose level in your blood. Insulin rings the bell on your cell walls to announce the presence of glucose outside. The cell then has to mobilize transporters from its interior to come to the wall, create an opening, and accept a molecule of glucose to transport it to a location inside.

According to the insulin resistance theory, certain cells of the body "resist" the presence of insulin, do not release glucose transporters to accept glucose, and the glucose ends up in your blood.

I disagree with this theory. Through my research, I have recognized that there is a better explanation for how high blood sugar happens. My idea, "the fatty acid burn theory," is far more logical and makes better biological sense. In the chapters that follow, I will explain to you the real cause of high blood sugar. I have kept these explanations as simple as possible, with many illustrations. This science is not as complicated as you might think. Give it a try. The more you understand, the smarter you will be at preventing diabetes in your life.

The following "illustrated story" will help you begin to understand my theory. Review it again after you finish the remaining chapters in Part 1.

[1]Joslin EP. Arteriosclerosis and diabetes. Ann Clin Med. 1927;5:1061

THE
REAL CAUSE
OF
DIABETES

THE
FATTY ACID
BURN THEORY

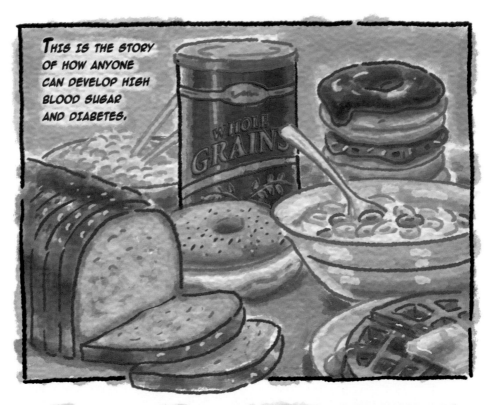

THIS IS THE STORY OF HOW ANYONE CAN DEVELOP HIGH BLOOD SUGAR AND DIABETES.

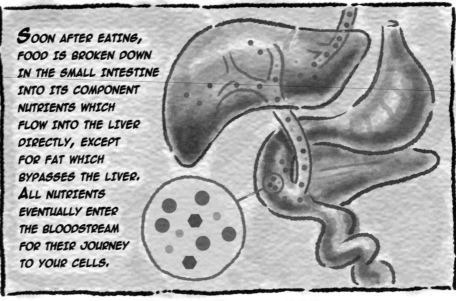

SOON AFTER EATING, FOOD IS BROKEN DOWN IN THE SMALL INTESTINE INTO ITS COMPONENT NUTRIENTS WHICH FLOW INTO THE LIVER DIRECTLY, EXCEPT FOR FAT WHICH BYPASSES THE LIVER. ALL NUTRIENTS EVENTUALLY ENTER THE BLOODSTREAM FOR THEIR JOURNEY TO YOUR CELLS.

Glucose Amino Acids Misc. Nutrients

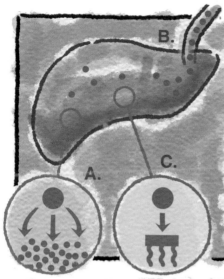

B.

A. **C.**

In the liver, glucose from the food you eat can be processed in 3 ways: (A) some is converted to glycogen for storage in the liver; (B) some is released into the bloodstream; and (C) the excess is converted into triglycerides, composed of three fatty acid molecules and one glycerol molecule. The liver sends the triglycerides to your fat cells for storage.

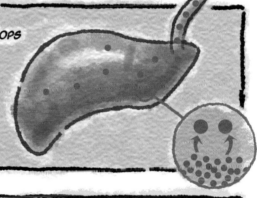

When your blood sugar drops between meals, the liver reconverts glycogen into glucose and releases it into the bloodstream for cells to burn for energy

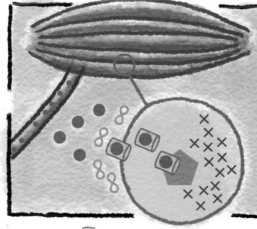

Ordinarily, when glucose arrives at muscle cells, insulin attracts glucose transporters in the cell to open a channel for glucose to enter. Muscles use the glucose to manufacture ATP, the source of energy for its cellular functions.

Glucose Transporter   Triglyerides   ATP   Mitochondria   Insulin

IN FAT CELLS, AN ENZYME CALLED LIPASE EXISTS OUTSIDE THE CELL (EXTERNAL LIPASE) AND INSIDE THE CELL (INTERNAL LIPASE). TRIGLYCERIDES ARRIVING AT A FAT CELL ARE TOO BIG TO ENTER. INSULIN ACTIVATES THE EXTERNAL LIPASE WHICH BREAKS THE TRIGLYCERIDE INTO 3 FATTY ACIDS AND 1 GLYCEROL. FATTY ACIDS ENTER THE CELL, WHERE THEY ARE COMBINED WITH A NEW GLYCEROL TO FORM TRIGLYCERIDE THAT IS STORED. INSULIN INHIBITS THE INTERNAL LIPASE FROM RELEASING THE FATTY ACIDS BACK INTO THE BLOOD STREAM.

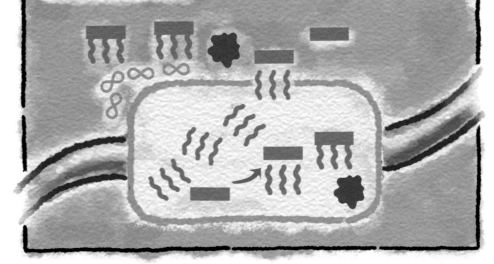

BETWEEN MEALS OR DURING EXERCISE, WHEN MUSCLES NEED MORE ENERGY, THE INTERNAL LIPASE IN FAT CELLS WILL BEGIN BREAKING DOWN STORED TRIGLYCERIDES INTO THEIR COMPONENT FATTY ACIDS. THESE CAN EXIT THE FAT CELL INTO THE BLOODSTREAM AND GO TO MUSCLE CELLS WHICH CAN BURN THEM FOR ENERGY INSTEAD OF GLUCOSE.

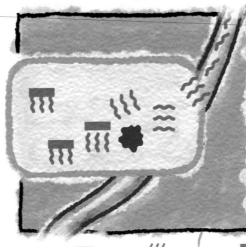

Glycerol   Fatty Acids in cell   Triglyerides   Insulin   Lipase   Fat Cell

THE INSULIN RESISTANCE THEORY CLAIMS THAT THE LIVER RELEASES GLUCOSE, MUSCLES DON'T ACCEPT GLUCOSE, AND FAT CELLS RELEASE FATTY ACIDS, ALL IN THE PRESENCE OF INSULIN. THIS THEORY IS NOT CORRECT.

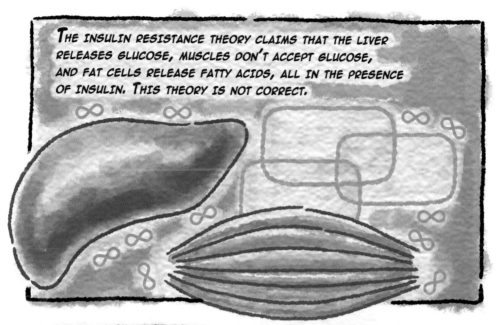

HERE IS THE REAL STORY OF HOW DIABETES HAPPENS. OVER TIME, IF YOU FILL YOUR FAT CELLS, THEY CAN NO LONGER ACCEPT TRIGLYCERIDES TRANSPORTED FROM THE LIVER. WHEN NEW TRIGLYCERIDES ARRIVE, THEY ARE CONVERTED TO FATTY ACIDS BY EXTERNAL LIPASE, BUT THERE IS NO ROOM FOR THEM IN THE FAT CELL. THE FATTY ACIDS SIMPLY GO BACK INTO THE BLOODSTREAM.

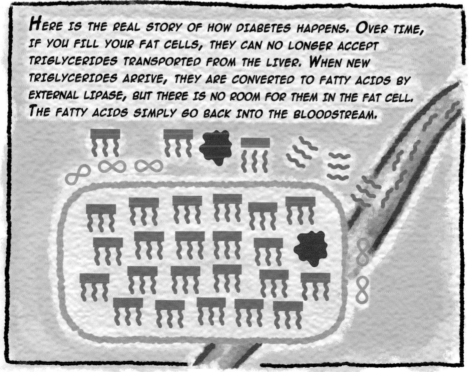

DUE TO THE FACT THAT YOUR BLOODSTREAM NOW HAS LARGE AMOUNTS OF FATTY ACIDS FLOWING THROUGH IT, YOUR LIVER BEGINS DEGRADING THEM INTO MOLECULES CALLED ACETYL COENZYME A. THESE ARE PACKAGED AS SMALL FATTY ACIDS AND RELEASED INTO THE BLOODSTREAM WHICH TRANSPORTS THEM RAPIDLY THROUGHOUT THE BODY.

WHEN YOUR BLOOD HAS A LOT OF CIRCULATING SMALL FATTY ACIDS, THE BRAIN RELEASES GROWTH HORMONE TO INSTRUCT MUSCLES TO CHANGE THEIR FUEL PREFERENCE FROM GLUCOSE TO FATTY ACIDS. MUSCLE CELLS HAVE NO MORE ROOM OR NEED FOR GLUCOSE. EVEN IN THE PRESENCE OF INSULIN, GLUCOSE TRANSPORTERS STAY IN THEIR HOLDING AREA. GLUCOSE THAT CANNOT ENTER THE CELL STAYS IN THE BLOODSTREAM. THIS IS THE MAIN CAUSE OF BLOOD SUGAR ELEVATION.

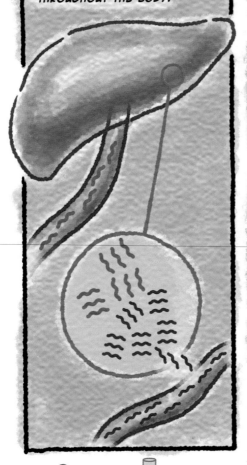

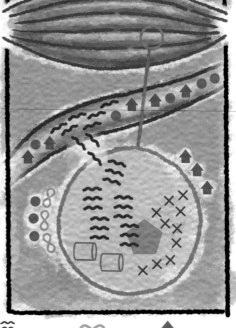

● Glucose   ⬭ Glucose Transporter   ≋ Small Fatty Acids   ∞ Insulin   ⬆ Growth Hormone

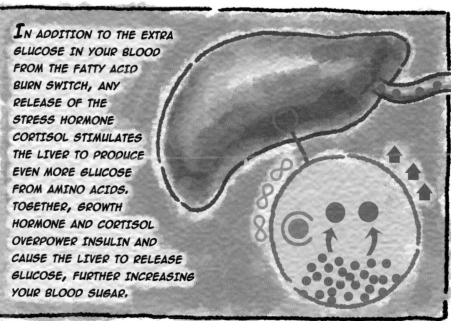

IN ADDITION TO THE EXTRA GLUCOSE IN YOUR BLOOD FROM THE FATTY ACID BURN SWITCH, ANY RELEASE OF THE STRESS HORMONE CORTISOL STIMULATES THE LIVER TO PRODUCE EVEN MORE GLUCOSE FROM AMINO ACIDS. TOGETHER, GROWTH HORMONE AND CORTISOL OVERPOWER INSULIN AND CAUSE THE LIVER TO RELEASE GLUCOSE, FURTHER INCREASING YOUR BLOOD SUGAR.

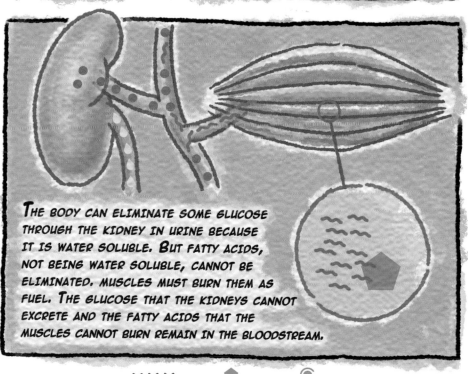

THE BODY CAN ELIMINATE SOME GLUCOSE THROUGH THE KIDNEY IN URINE BECAUSE IT IS WATER SOLUBLE. BUT FATTY ACIDS, NOT BEING WATER SOLUBLE, CANNOT BE ELIMINATED. MUSCLES MUST BURN THEM AS FUEL. THE GLUCOSE THAT THE KIDNEYS CANNOT EXCRETE AND THE FATTY ACIDS THAT THE MUSCLES CANNOT BURN REMAIN IN THE BLOODSTREAM.

 ATP   Mitochondria   Cortisol

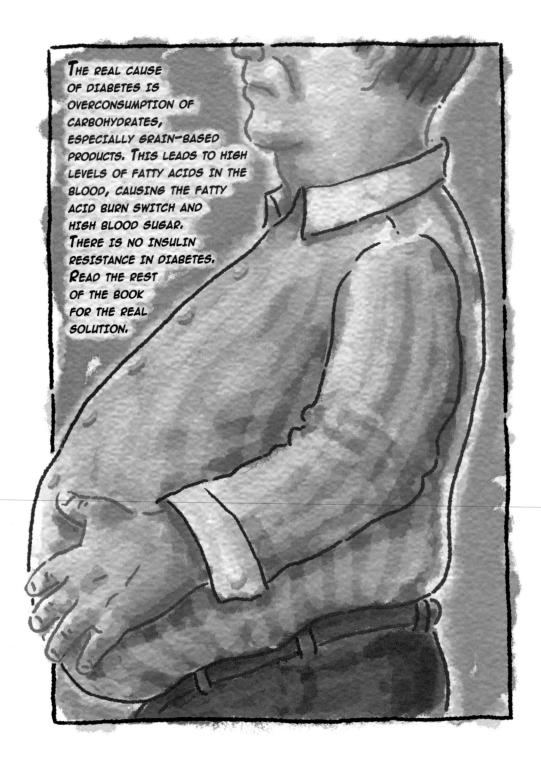

THE REAL CAUSE OF DIABETES IS OVERCONSUMPTION OF CARBOHYDRATES, ESPECIALLY GRAIN-BASED PRODUCTS. THIS LEADS TO HIGH LEVELS OF FATTY ACIDS IN THE BLOOD, CAUSING THE FATTY ACID BURN SWITCH AND HIGH BLOOD SUGAR. THERE IS NO INSULIN RESISTANCE IN DIABETES. READ THE REST OF THE BOOK FOR THE REAL SOLUTION.

CHAPTER 3

The Current Theory about Type 2 Diabetes

The current medical theory for Type 2 diabetes is that it is related to insulin production or insulin resistance. In any literature on Type 2 diabetes, the theory is explained something like this:

> In Type 2 diabetes, your pancreas either does not produce enough insulin or your cells become resistant to the insulin produced. The result is high blood sugar (hyperglycemia) that leads to serious damage to many of the body's systems. If you have diabetes in your family, you are at risk for getting diabetes yourself. If you are of African-American, Latino, Native American, Polynesian, Micronesian, or Eskimo ancestry, your risk is higher. Losing weight is one of the most effective measures to prevent diabetes.

Like many people, you will probably find this explanation confusing. First, it mentions what seem to be two different reasons why Type 2 diabetes occurs: 1) your pancreas is not producing enough insulin, or 2) your body's cells become resistant to insulin and therefore cannot absorb the glucose in your bloodstream.

It is difficult to understand which cause could be the culprit if you have been told you are prediabetic or already have diabetes. If you don't have diabetes but are worried about getting it, you probably have no idea what you can do to prevent insulin resistance from occurring or your pancreas from producing insufficient insulin.

Worse, no matter which of these explanations your doctor gives you or which one you tend to believe, neither makes complete sense. It might be logical to think that the pancreas can wear out over time and fail to produce enough insulin or that cells can become resistant to insulin over time, but why doesn't this happen to almost everyone? We're all human and we all age, right? Diabetes should be far more widespread if this were true.

Furthermore, if losing weight prevents diabetes, why don't all overweight and obese people get diabetes? If genetics is a factor in developing diabetes, why don't all children of a parent with diabetes inherit it? How is it that one sibling gets diabetes but not another? And why are people from certain ethnic groups more at risk?

The biggest question for me as a medical doctor is: What research exists that proves people with Type 2 diabetes do not produce enough insulin or that their cells have become resistant to it?

I hope you agree that these are all important questions, to which medical science has yet to provide good answers. Let me walk you through each of the insulin theories and explain why they are likely incorrect, despite their long-term acceptance in the medical community.

A Side Trip to the Pancreas First

Before we discuss the first theory, it is important to learn about the organ called the pancreas, as it is the key player in both of these theories. The pancreas sits behind the stomach in the upper abdomen. It has two main functions, an *endocrine* function and an *exocrine* function. The *endocrine* function means it secretes two hormones the body needs to regulate blood sugar. One hormone is *insulin*, which helps reduce glucose in the blood. The other is *glucagon* and has the opposite function of elevating the blood glucose concentration. The *exocrine* function of the pancreas means that it secretes digestive enzymes used in the small intestine to further break down the carbohydrates, proteins and lipids (fats) in the foods we eat.

We are now ready to examine the two theories.

The Inadequate Production of Insulin Theory

This theory is based on the suspicion that the pancreas stops producing an adequate supply of insulin to help the high levels of glucose in your bloodstream get into cells. When you were a child and teenager, and even in your 20s or 30s, the pancreas produced adequate amounts of insulin, but for unknown reasons, the theory says that at some point for many adults, the pancreas fails to secrete enough.

One of the conjectures of the theory of insufficient production is that the condition worsens over time. The rationale is that as glucose mounts in the blood, the pancreas secretes more and more insulin, causing it to begin functioning on overdrive as it attempts to secrete ever-larger amounts to make up for the deficit. Eventually, the pancreatic cells that secrete insulin reach a point of fatigue and stop producing much at all. They wear out, like the parts of a car engine that has gone too many miles.

The above explanation might make sense if we accept two facts. First, every organ in the body is designed to have an adequate number of cells to last a lifetime. However, if an organ is tasked to work overtime for a long period, it may become exhausted and unable to function well. The elevation of the glucose level in your blood is one of the surest means to overstimulate the pancreas to manufacture and release insulin beyond its normal capacity. So this wearing out could be true.

Second, every organ in the body is limited in what it can do even under the strongest stimulus. For example, there is an upper limit to the volume of air your lungs can accept when you exercise to your maximum capability. There is also a limit to the number of beats your heart can generate to sustain adequate blood supply when you exercise to your maximum capacity. In the case of the pancreas, its inability to meet the demand for insulin might reflect that you have reached the natural limit of what this organ can achieve. Expecting the pancreas to keep secreting more and more insulin would be like squeezing an orange or a lemon after it is dry but expecting it to keep releasing more juice.

A blood test, the c-peptide test, is used to detect if someone is not producing enough insulin. If the test is positive, the person is usually prescribed, as a first step, oral medication (pills) that stimulate the pancreas to produce more insulin. If a person's insulin production is extremely low, or if it becomes low after oral medication is used for a period of time, the person is often prescribed insulin injections. These are self-administered in the form of a small pen-like device with a needle at its tip that the patient inserts directly into the skin of the abdomen following a meal. A dial on the device can determine how much insulin is injected under the skin to compensate for the inadequate supply produced by the person's pancreas.

While this theory may seem logical and can be verified using insulin testing, it does not answer many questions:

- What caused the initial insufficient production at this specific time in the person's lifetime?
- Why do some people develop insufficient insulin production and not others?
- Can pancreatic fatigue be reversed such that adequate natural insulin secretion can resume?
- Can doctors detect when someone is about to go into pancreatic overdrive and prevent it from happening?
- Can forcing the pancreatic cells with medication to produce more insulin exhaust them earlier than they would otherwise have become exhausted?

Despite the prevalence of Type 2 diabetes, there has been very little medical research on these issues. The lack of clear answers to the above questions suggests that the theory of pancreatic dysfunction as the causative factor in Type 2 diabetes is open to question.

The Insulin Resistance Theory

In this theory about Type 2 diabetes, there are adequate levels of insulin in the blood, but for some reason the insulin hormone does not perform normally and fails to channel glucose into cells. In the prediabetic phase (usually associated with excess weight gain), blood insulin levels rise above accepted normal ranges both when the person has been fasting and after eating food. Blood glucose levels may have been normal when the person was younger, but as the person ages there is a fasting or post-food rise in blood glucose, despite the elevated insulin levels. Why does this happen?

The explanation most often given is that the body's cells start to "resist" the presence of insulin to let glucose in. No matter how much insulin there is, blood sugar remains high. However, medical science is not yet able to explain why this resistance occurs or what the mechanism of it is.

One of the most curious, if not suspicious, aspects of this theory is that it recognizes that insulin resistance does not occur in all the body's cells. There are only three main groups of cells where insulin resistance is thought to occur: 1) muscle cells that have not been warmed up (inactive muscle cells), 2) the liver, and 3) fat cells.

As mentioned earlier, active exercising muscle does not need the assistance of insulin to let glucose enter the muscle cells. However, when muscle cells have been resting, the insulin resistance theory claims that there is a sharp reduction in the amount of glucose that diffuses into the cells in relationship to how much glucose remains in the blood after eating. This is considered to be evidence that the muscle cells have become resistant to the action of insulin through some type of faulty internal mechanism.

It is also thought that the liver becomes resistant to insulin because in Type 2 diabetes, the liver continues to release glucose from glycogen even when the bloodstream is already overflowing with glucose. Remember that glycogen is broken down when the body needs glucose. As mentioned, insulin normally blocks the liver from converting glycogen to glucose. Thus, it is theorized that the liver cells also become resistant to insulin's effects because they keep producing glucose from glycogen.

As for fat cells, here is what the theory proposes regarding their supposed resistance to insulin. First, triglyceride produced in the liver is brought by the blood to fat tissue for storage. The triglyceride molecule is too large to enter the fat cell. An enzyme called *lipase* resides *outside* the fat cell, which insulin activates to break down the triglyceride molecules into their component fatty acids.

These are small enough to enter the fat cell. Once inside, the fatty acids combine with a glycerol molecule manufactured from glucose inside the fat cell and are reconstituted into triglyceride for storage in the fat cell (figure 7).

Later, when the body needs extra energy, another lipase enzyme, which resides *inside* the fat cell, breaks the stored triglyceride back down into fatty acids that exit out of the fat cell into the bloodstream, where they can be used by muscle cells. Ordinarily, insulin inhibits this lipase enzyme, preventing the release of fatty acids from stored triglyceride (figure 8).

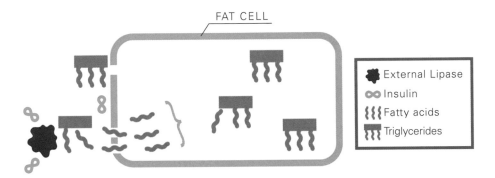

Figure 7. Triglyceride produced in the liver arriving at a fat cell is too large to enter. Insulin activates external lipase outside the fat cell to break the triglyceride molecules into fatty acids that can enter the cell. Inside, these fatty acids are reconstituted into triglyceride for storage.

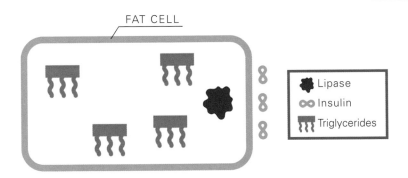

Figure 8. Normally the presence of insulin prevents internal lipase from releasing fatty acids from triglycerides.

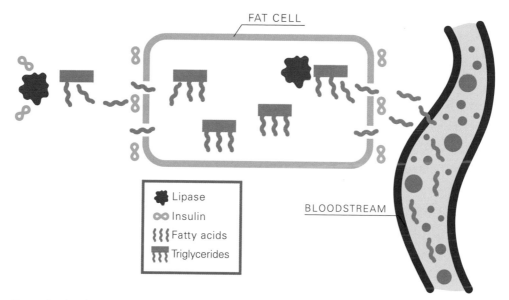

Figure 9. The Theory of Insulin Resistance in Fat Cells
The insulin resistance theory claims that insulin triggers external lipase (left) to break down triglycerides into fatty acids that can enter the fat cell. But the theory also claims that internal lipase is resistant to insulin and allows fatty acids to exit the fat cell and go into the bloodstream, even when insulin is present. How is it possible for only one of the two identical enzymes to be resistant while the other is not?

According to the insulin resistance theory, however, it is thought that something goes wrong with this process. Large amounts of fatty acids are released from fat tissue, even in the presence of insulin. It is currently accepted that of the two fat cell-associated lipase enzymes, both of which perform identical functions, only the internal lipase shows resistance to the presence of insulin while the outside lipase responds normally (figure 9). This is considered why people with Type 2 diabetes have high levels of fatty acids in their blood.

The above theory might be understandable based on how the body normally uses fatty acids. The total amount of energy stored as carbohydrate in the body is less than 1000 calories, while each pound of fat packs 3500 calories. Therefore, it is advantageous for the body to facilitate burning fatty acids from stored fat to produce energy rather than glucose. This is what happens naturally in the biggest consumer of glucose for energy, your muscle cells. The amount of ATP and glucose stored inside muscles provide enough fuel to last only a few minutes. Muscles are programmed to switch to burning fatty acids when any muscle activity lasts longer than several minutes. This conserves at least some glucose stored in the muscles so it can be used when the cycle starts again with the next activity. When the extended activity is over, the muscles normally switch back to using glucose to produce ATP.

But why don't the muscles of people with prediabetes or diabetes switch back to glucose for ATP energy production? The resistance of internal lipase to insulin is the usual explanation for why this doesn't occur. While insulin should block the further release of fatty acids out of fat cells, the theory posits that the resistance of lipase to insulin allows fatty acids to exit fat cells and flow into muscle cells, preventing the switch back to glucose. However, the mechanism by which internal lipase resists insulin while external lipase responds to it normally has not been identified. The theory is illogical.

Why the Insulin Resistance Theory is Questionable

I have examined the insulin resistance theory in depth for years, and have concluded that it doesn't make biological sense. Proof of this is evident if we examine many related mechanisms of the body that should suffer or be altered if insulin resistance were true. Let's review these anomalies that demonstrate how insulin resistance cannot explain the cause of Type 2 diabetes.

1. No loss of the body's ability to regulate heat

If the millions of cells in the body were resistant to insulin, particularly in our muscle tissue, we would expect the body to have great difficulty regulating its consistent internal temperature, 98.6 degrees Fahrenheit. Let me explain why this would happen.

The body is like a home furnace that burns glucose to produce heat. Under normal conditions, the temperature of the inner core of the human body remains constant within ±1 degree Fahrenheit 24 hours a day. Even when the outside air temperature ranges from a low of 55 degrees Fahrenheit below zero to a high of 130 degrees Fahrenheit, the body still maintains an almost constant internal core body temperature. In contrast to our core temperature, our skin temperature can rise and fall with the temperature of the surroundings.

Where does the body get this internal heat? In babies, specialized fat cells containing "brown fat" generate heat mainly to warm major blood vessels that supply the brain with blood. Cells storing brown fat are different from regular fat cells by virtue of their ability to produce heat instead of ATP molecules in their mitochondria. The survival of rodents during exposure to cold temperature is a testament to the ability of their brown fat cells to keep them warm. Brown fat cells play a much smaller role in warming the human body, especially in adults who have reduced amounts of brown fat.

In adults, we get our heat from the many metabolic activities occurring inside each cell. As you learned, ATP, which is made from glucose molecules, is the ready source of energy in every living cell. Many calories of energy may be contained in each ATP molecule, but only a few are needed for the molecular reactions in the cell. The remainder of the energy created when ATP decomposes is distributed in the body in the form of heat, just as your entire kitchen heats up when you are cooking in the oven.

Even under the best of conditions, only 30 percent of the energy from food is used for metabolic functions of the body. The excess heat from each cell contributes to maintaining your body's core temperature. Highly active organs such as the liver, brain, heart and skeletal muscles produce most of the heat in the body. It's amazing that the core body temperature is kept within a very narrow range with contributions from trillions of tiny furnaces.

Given that about 40 percent of the body is skeletal muscle which consumes 80 to 90 percent of the glucose from your food, it is clear that muscle activity contributes a significant amount of the heat used to maintain the body temperature. But here's exactly the proof that insulin resistance is not a valid theory. If muscle cells supposedly cannot utilize glucose as fuel because of insulin resistance, then maintaining our body temperature would be significantly impaired. However, there is no evidence of impaired body temperature maintenance in individuals with Type 2 diabetes.

One might argue against this proof, claiming that perhaps other parts of the body compensate for impaired glucose-generated heat production in muscle cells. Perhaps other organs begin to function at a higher level to produce enough heat to compensate for the loss of heat from muscles resistant to insulin. But if this were true, we should see evidence of increased activity of the involved organs and systems contributing to the maintenance of body temperature.

But we don't see such evidence. No other body organ has been found to be extra active and no byproduct of activity from other organs has been detected in excess of normal in individuals with Type 2 diabetes. Increased metabolic activity leading to greater heat production in organs other than muscle has not been found.

In short, it does not seem that insulin resistance can explain why our muscles continue to function and even generate the heat our body needs to maintain its constant temperature, nor do we see other organs compensating for a lack of muscle-powered heat. Our muscles continue to derive energy even while glucose is not getting into them. (Keep this point in mind, as it is a key point in my alternative theory. Our muscles are deriving energy from something and don't need the glucose. We'll return to this point shortly.)

2. No loss of muscle strength

If insulin resistance prevented muscles from using as much glucose, we should see evidence of a weakening of muscle function, just as you would expect an automobile to function poorly if the engine's ability to burn gasoline was impaired.

A muscle consists of fibers that are made of protein filaments. When muscle fibers contract, one type of protein filament pulls itself over another, similar to a person climbing up a dangling rope using both arms. While some "arms" of the protein filament are gripping, others relax. The addition of ATP is essential for the "arms" to relax, so that they have the energy for the next grip. (The most extreme example of what happens when there is no ATP to make muscle fibers relax is "rigor mortis," the state of contracture that occurs after death.)

This suggests that if the main source of ATP is glucose metabolism, the absence of glucose due to insulin resistance should prevent muscle fibers from relaxing. However, diabetes does not prevent people from running, jumping, lifting heavy boxes, dancing, skiing, or walking. Type 2 diabetics are often aging seniors who are losing muscle mass, but not at rates faster than the general population of seniors. There is no evidence of progressive weakening of muscle power or deterioration of muscle function in individuals with decades long Type 2 diabetes, even if they required increasing doses of medications including insulin to regulate their blood sugar levels. In short, it seems unlikely that insulin resistance prevents muscles from obtaining energy, even if it is not facilitating the entry of glucose.

3. No loss of triglyceride production in the liver

Some medical scientists have suggested that the liver is the first organ to show resistance to insulin. Given that insulin normally *restricts* glucose production in the liver, a person with Type 2 diabetes with insulin resistance should produce lots of glucose in the liver (since the insulin is not working to restrict it). The scientific evidence to support this claim is the fact that, in people with Type 2 diabetes who are fasting—and thus not consuming carbohydrates—we do see a rise of blood glucose proportionate to glucose production in the liver.

But let me counter this argument. When more carbohydrates are consumed than can be used for immediate energy, insulin normally promotes the conversion of excess glucose into fatty acids in the liver. These fatty acids are subsequently converted to triglycerides and transported in the blood to fat cells for storage. If the liver becomes resistant to insulin, however, triglyceride formation in the liver should be correspondingly reduced. Yet the level of circulating triglycerides is higher than normal when a Type 2 diabetic person exhibits an elevated glucose level in the blood. How does it happen that insulin resistance causes both high glucose production AND high triglyceride production, two mutually exclusive processes?

It could be argued that the finding of increased glucose production and high triglyceride formation in the liver at the same time occurs because *only part of the liver* is resistant to the action of insulin. But there are no observations to explain why different parts of the liver would react differently to the presence of insulin. There are also no observations explaining how this is sustained throughout the life of this condition in someone with Type 2 diabetes.

4. No finding of any agents that block insulin

With many diseases, an agent such as an antibody is sometimes found to block the utilization of molecules in cells. Given this pattern in the body, insulin resistance might be considered the result of such an agent blocking the attachment of insulin to its receptor on the cell surface. Yet no one has discovered or demonstrated an agent that blocks the binding of insulin with the insulin receptor on cells at the time Type 2 diabetes is diagnosed.

5. No proof that changes in cells cause a failure to recognize the presence of insulin

Some might suggest that resistance to insulin could occur because the cells that should respond to the presence of insulin outside them do not do so. Or, perhaps some event has occurred in the cell to negate its response to insulin, such as a change in the manufacture and movement of modules needed to transport glucose inside the cell.

However, here again there is no evidence of fluctuations in the number of insulin receptors or a lower level of function in the insulin-resistant organs corresponding to the fluctuating levels of insulin.

6. No other cells of the body appear to develop insulin resistance

It is known that every type of body cell needs glucose to function. It is also known that some cells vary in the type of specialized glucose transport modules within them that have different degrees of affinity for glucose and use different transport mechanisms. For example, glucose transporters in red blood cells are different from those in cells in the kidney, lining of the intestine, the liver, and pancreatic cells that produce insulin. Nerve cells have their own glucose transporters. Cells of the fat tissue, heart and skeletal muscle have a different type of glucose transporter.

One could say that these different types of glucose transporters are why insulin resistance is thought to occur in only three types of cells: muscle, fat, and liver cells. However, this has never been shown and is illogical. Insulin acts on receptors on the exterior cell wall of all cells, and its mechanism of functioning has never been proven to differ among the many types of cells. Regardless of the type of transporter used inside, insulin is nothing more than a messenger to call the transporters into action. In addition, several types of cells have the same transporters as muscle, fat, and liver cells and they are not insulin resistant.

In short, it is illogical to say that insulin resistance of only certain cells in the body is the causative factor of Type 2 diabetes. This cannot be accepted unless a reason and/or mechanism by which other cells avoid becoming insulin resistant can be identified and proven.

The Only Logical Conclusion: Insulin Resistance is Incorrect

All the above arguments point to gaping holes in the theory of insulin resistance as the cause of Type 2 diabetes. To date, there is absolutely no proof that insulin resistance accurately explains why the body's cells do not intake glucose the way they normally do. In addition to the six anomalies I raised above, many other questions need to be answered before insulin resistance can be accepted as the causative mechanism of Type 2 diabetes, including:

- Why would the body suddenly develop resistance to the action of one of its own hormones?
- Why do sensitive cells only target insulin as the hormone they are resistant to when there are other hormones they could also be resistant to?
- Is the biology behind such a development the same in all individuals who become diabetic, whether they are obese, thin, young or pregnant?

Furthermore, we have no information on whether the cause of resistance and the mechanism by which it occurs are the same in all affected cells—skeletal muscle, the liver and fat cells. In the absence of an obvious biological mechanism to explain how resistance occurs, it is scientifically unsound to claim that these three types of cells are the only organs in Type 2 diabetes afflicted with insulin resistance.

KEY POINTS

- The insulin theory of diabetes actually proposes two concepts: 1) that the pancreas stops producing enough insulin and eventually becomes worn out trying to produce more, and 2) certain cells of the body—the liver, muscle cells, and fat cells—become resistant to the presence of insulin.

- The first concept could be plausible, but why don't other organs of the body wear out? And why doesn't insufficient production happen to all or most people?

- The second concept might make sense, also, but there is no proof for how insulin resistance occurs or why it happens in just three body tissues. There is also no explanation for why the liver produces both high amounts of glucose and high amounts of triglycerides, two mutually exclusive processes.

CHAPTER 4

Faulty Research on Insulin Resistance

I would like to suggest that the insulin resistance theory is based on a biased interpretation of research studies rather than on science based on evidence and facts.

The most noted of these research studies is a test done with what is called a hyperinsulinemic-euglycemic clamp.[1] The test, which is conducted in a lab, is designed to measure the *sensitivity* of the liver to insulin. For the test, insulin is infused at a constant rate and glucose is infused at variable rates into the vein of a subject. The rate of glucose infusion is adjusted to maintain a specific blood glucose level, depending on how much glucose the liver is producing. If the liver is producing a large amount of glucose, less of it is infused in the subject, and vice versa.

From this test, it has been determined that a diabetic liver appears to be insulin resistant because it continues to produce glucose even when glucose is being infused into the subject. (Recall that insulin is supposed to prevent the liver cells

---

[1] Hyperinsulinemic-Euglycemic Clamp to Assess Insulin Sensitivity In Vivo. Chapter 15. Methods in Molecular Biology, vol. 560. C. Stocker (ed.), Humana Press. 2009

from producing glucose.) Radioactive-labeled glucose is used to calculate the uptake of glucose by muscles and fat tissue.

However, while this test may prove that the liver continues to produce glucose even in the presence of insulin, it does not explain why muscle cells do not accept glucose into their cell walls, despite the presence of insulin. It is true that cells do not open channels to welcome glucose inside, but this does not prove that the cells are barring glucose from entering. There is a disconnect going on here since the actual insulin resistance has not been measured. There could be other reasons why glucose is not entering muscle cells. In other words, the test still does not get to the root of why or how our cells reject glucose.

Nevertheless, experts in diabetes always present this test as the gold-standard method of proving the existence of *resistance* to insulin. This is similar to conducting tests to determine a person's emotional intelligence and presenting that score as that of their intelligence quotient (IQ). The two tests may be similar, but they prove different things.

Let me present a different analogy to explain what might be happening in cells. Imagine a busy restaurant in which patrons keep coming in, even though the place is full. They all wait patiently in the vestibule. They usually don't attribute the delay in getting their table to the host or hostess simply refusing to seat them, but to the obvious fact that all the tables are already taken. Once the patrons know the *why* (all tables are taken), the *how* (not opening the door to the dining room) becomes self-explanatory. The host has nothing to do with it—the dining room is simply full.

This could be happening in our cells when it comes to insulin and glucose. New glucose arrives, but the cell is already creating energy and does not need any more. Since cells need energy for survival, there has to be a reason they are refusing the admission of glucose when both insulin and glucose are present outside the cell wall. That reason is the cells are already burning something else for fuel—fatty acids. This is what my theory proposes is happening. We will examine this in detail in the next chapters.

A Theory Full of Holes

This insulin resistance theory is full of inconsistencies and challenges that make its accuracy suspect. Without any means to understand the mechanism of insulin resistance, to identify the precise cellular locations where it occurs, or to measure the degree of insulin resistance, doctors are left to speculate on the efficacy of different treatment modalities to control blood sugar levels. As mentioned, the c-peptide test can be used to measure the progressive reduction in insulin secretion in patients with long-lasting Type 2 diabetes, but there is no test that measures *insulin resistance* in a person such that its actual severity can be graded and dealt with. (Some diabetes specialists consider high blood glucose after fasting or post food combined with elevated insulin levels as a test that proves insulin resistance, but again, the proof is only indirect.)

Having an insulin resistance test could help doctors identify a range of normal values so we could assess when the prediabetes condition might be starting to occur, or whether it is worsening in someone with Type 2 diabetes despite treatment. Such a test might also allow a patient who has maintained normal blood sugar levels for at least five years through diet and lifestyle modifications to feel reassured that they have been cured of the illness. The lack of a test impacts most every decision about treating Type 2 diabetes, including:

- how to determine the best type of medical therapy based on the degree of insulin resistance,
- how to change or add medications during treatment,
- how to assess a patient's response to the treatment, and
- how to determine the duration of treatment.

We know that weight loss leads to rapid reduction in blood glucose levels in overweight diabetic individuals. This effect is supposed to occur in part because it is believed that weight loss leads to an improved response to insulin in tissues. But without a test to measure the initial degree of insulin resistance and to determine in which cells it occurs, we are left to guess which cells suddenly become more responsive to insulin.

Similarly, we know that physical exercise is often correlated with less muscle resistance to insulin—or at least to muscle cells accepting glucose. But again, without a test, how can this be verified?

Finally, due to the progressive nature of Type 2 diabetes, insulin therapy is prescribed for many patients, but without calculating the relative contributions of the patient's possible insulin deficiency versus insulin resistance.[2] In addition, no mechanism has been proposed explaining how cells supposedly resistant to insulin become less resistant when there is more insulin outside due to the medication.

In short, insulin resistance should be considered an interesting hypothesis that attempts to explain the cause of elevated blood sugar. But like the ancient astronomical theory that the sun revolves around the earth, when the facts do not support a hypothesis, it is time to seek out a new explanation based on better observations and a more accurate medical understanding.

KEY POINT

- The gold standard test purporting to prove insulin resistance does not measure insulin resistance.

[2] Executive Summary: Standards of Medical Care in Diabetes—Diabetes Care, Volume 37, S5-S13, American Diabetes Association. January 2014

CHAPTER 5

A Smarter Theory for the Cause of Type 2 Diabetes

Let's begin by talking about how glucose is regulated in "normal" people, including prediabetics who are in control of their blood sugar.

In these individuals, blood glucose is finely regulated to stay between 60-140 mg/dl and seldom rises above 140 mg/dl (milligrams per deciliter). This means they can accommodate normal and even occasionally high levels of ingested glucose into their cells. They have normal energy stores, and occasionally above-normal stores until that energy is used. Their ability to regulate glucose protects the body against the untoward effects of *hyperglycemia* (too much glucose). When this occurs, the abundance of glucose (higher than 180 mg/dl) forces the kidneys to rid the body of the excess through frequent urination. The loss of so much body water causes short-term dehydration in diabetics. The long-term effect of excessive glucose in the blood is that the molecules attach themselves to different proteins, affecting their functions and leading to complications such as nerve or kidney damage.

Why can't a patient with Type 2 diabetes occasionally dispose of excess glucose and store fat in fat cells like in normal people? Why can't skeletal muscle, fat tissue, and the liver transport the excess glucose into their cells for storage like in normal people? Could there be a different explanation for high blood sugar than reduced insulin secretion from the pancreas or insulin resistance?

These questions prompted me to seek an alternative theory about the cause of Type 2 diabetes.

On the Hunt for a New Theory of Insufficient Insulin Production

A common and widely accepted practice in medical science is to test a concept presented as a causative factor in human illness first in animals before treatments are formulated. For example, a virus suspected of causing an illness in humans can be injected into an animal. The animal can then be observed for symptoms of the illness affiliated with the virus.

To understand the illness called diabetes, animals have been injected with chemicals that destroy specific pancreatic cells that produce insulin. These animals showed signs and symptoms similar to those predicted when insulin-producing cells are killed. However, these findings are identical to the illness in humans called Type 1 diabetes (also called juvenile-onset diabetes), in which the pancreatic cells that produce insulin are destroyed by cells of the immune system. As a result, the body cannot produce insulin at all.

In a person who is prediabetic or has Type 2 diabetes, pancreatic cells that produce insulin do not show evidence of structural destruction. The cells appear normal and seem to be able to function normally. However, as mentioned before, one Type 2 diabetes theory asserts that pancreatic cells reduce their secretion of insulin in spite of intense and sustained stimulation. It does appear that the pancreas can recover on its own from this overstimulation and begin secreting insulin again. The evidence for this is that several medications are able to force the pancreas to secrete more insulin, at least for a while.

However, I feel that by looking at this explanation from a different perspective, we can come up with a better theory than the supposed reduced secretion of insulin in Type 2 diabetes. An analogy may help you understand the thesis I'm about to propose.

Imagine a hamburger restaurant capable of producing a maximum of 1000 hamburgers per hour. If customer demand is the same as the production capacity, the restaurant is functionally adequate. But suppose customer demand goes up by 200 and 1200 burgers per hour are now needed. It would be correct to say that the production has become inadequate to meet the demand. However, couldn't we also say that the restaurant is functioning at the capacity it was designed for?

By analogy, when someone consumes a lot of food, producing excessive glucose, we are tempted to conclude that insulin secretion is inadequate compared to the amount needed to move the higher volume of sugar out of the bloodstream. Yet, if you were to consider the amount of insulin the pancreas is expected to produce and release on a given day, it could very well be that insulin secretion is perfectly within its normal limits for that person. The pancreas is functioning to its capacity. It just appears to produce too little insulin to handle the amount of glucose in the blood. Medications that stimulate the pancreas to produce more insulin are simply forcing the organ to increase its capacity to produce insulin, not compensating for reduced production.

From this perspective, the secretion of insulin is sufficient. The problem is that the pancreas simply cannot keep up with the person's overconsumption of foods that generate glucose.

Why would the body allow such higher levels of glucose to occur in the blood in the first place? Why wouldn't the pancreas just increase the production of insulin on its own to match the higher levels of glucose in the blood, thereby preventing the rise of glucose to a harmful level?

One reason that the pancreas may produce only so much insulin could simply be self-preservation. By not responding to intense, temporary over-stimulations over the course of an entire lifetime, pancreatic cells that produce insulin can remain functionally active for a longer period of time. Your body is simply taking good care of itself, in the same way that you don't drive a car 200,000 miles per year and expect it to last a lifetime.

But I suggest there is also another, perhaps even more important reason for the pancreas to fail to increase its insulin production when glucose levels skyrocket, and that is to protect the command and control centers in the brain from glucose deprivation. If insulin secretion in the body rises any time there is a sudden elevation of blood glucose levels, glucose will be forced into all cells throughout the body even if they don't need it. Then, as the blood sugar falls rapidly, insulin secretion would also sharply decrease. This risks dramatic swings in insulin production that could lead to a "timing mismatch" between production of insulin and the blood sugar levels. One result of such a timing mismatch could be *hypoglycemia*, too little blood sugar, which deprives the nerve cells in the brain of glucose. This condition can severely affect mental functions, leading to mental imbalances and even coma. Thus, it would seem biologically sound for the brain to instruct the pancreas to produce insulin, but only up to a certain level.

On the Hunt for a New Theory to Replace Insulin Resistance

The section above explained that insufficient insulin production may simply be a relative matter. The pancreas produces enough insulin for normal and for occasional above-normal needs, but cannot match the insulin needs of excessive blood sugar that occur when people overconsume foods that convert into glucose. But what about the theory of insulin resistance? What might be an alternative explanation for this?

My answer, which I hinted at in the prior chapter, is that cells do not accept glucose because they don't need it. They are utilizing something else for energy—*fatty acids*. Insulin resistance is not preventing glucose from entering your cells. Rather, your muscle cells are rejecting glucose because they are already filled with fatty acids that they are using for fuel. In effect, the theory of insulin resistance is off the mark and has nothing to do with the metabolic process actually taking place to cause high blood sugar levels.

As you learned, your cells are like hybrid engines that can burn either glucose or fatty acids to fuel their energy needs. Generally, glucose is utilized first, but when fatty acids are readily available, they can also be used for energy. The question is, what triggers your cells to switch to burning fatty acids rather than glucose?

The switch happens in this way. First, if you are eating too much and producing too much glucose, your liver is also producing a lot of fatty acids that are derived from glucose. The triglycerides made out of fatty acids produced in your liver are sent through your bloodstream to your body's fat cells, where they are stored. (Recall that triglyceride molecules are too big to enter, however, so a enzyme called *lipase* breaks them down into smaller fatty acids that enter the fat cells where they are reconstituted into triglycerides for storage.)

But as you continue to overeat or become less active, your body eventually fills up all your fat cells with triglycerides produced from the foods you ate. This occurs as you age and if you become more sedentary. The body also has stem cells that can become fat cells if needed. Once your normal fat cells are full, some of those stem cells turn into fat cells. As we all know, our bodies have a tendency to store fat in the tummy, thighs and butt, where most of the fat cells are located. You usually don't need scientific proof that you are consuming too much and producing too many triglycerides that are stored as body fat because all you need to do is weigh yourself or look in the mirror.

Genetics plays a direct role in your body's ability to store fat. Two children from the same parents can be different in their genetically-determined fat cell storage capacity, just as they can in their eye color or height. One can inherit stem cells to produce a lot of fat cells, and that child can become heavy or obese if he or she overeats. The other can inherit stem cells that create very few body fat cells, and that child remains thin for life, even if he or she overeats. However, both can become diabetic, so don't jump to conclusions that only fat people are prone to diabetes. We'll explain this shortly.

Fat cells are unlike muscle cells. Since they are primarily used for storage, not activity, they need very little glucose to produce energy to function. They do use some glucose to produce *glycerol*, the molecule needed to reconstitute triglyceride from the fatty acids that have entered the cells from the blood. But when the body's fat storage capacity is saturated, fat cells can no longer use any glucose or accept any more fatty acids. They are full to capacity. The implications of this are critical in helping us recognize why blood sugar rises and how it is has nothing to do with insulin resistance.

How the Switch to Burning Fatty Acids Occurs

When fat cells are full and do not need any glucose, it stays in the bloodstream, increasing your blood sugar. There is another consequence of having all the fat cells in your body filled to capacity: *you now have an abundance of fatty acids flowing in your bloodstream.*

The insulin resistance theory claims that the internal lipase in your fat cells is resistant to insulin and therefore continues its work of releasing fatty acids from inside fat cells in spite of the presence of insulin, which should normally cause this process to shut down. But my theory explains the metabolic activity much more logically, as it makes no sense that *external* lipase responds to insulin while *internal* lipase shows resistance.

What is actually happening is that your fat cells are not resistant to insulin at all. Insulin does indeed stimulate the outside lipase, which acts on the triglycerides outside fat cells to break them down into fatty acids. These fatty acids would normally enter the fat cells where they can be reconstituted into triglycerides, along with the help of the glucose that has entered the cell. But since your fat cells are already full, they cannot accommodate any more of the fatty acid molecules. Instead, what happens is that almost immediately after the triglycerides outside the fat cells have been broken into fatty acids, they are swept into the bloodstream. It is this abundance of fatty acids in your blood that triggers muscle cells to begin burning fatty acids rather than glucose (figures 10 and 11).

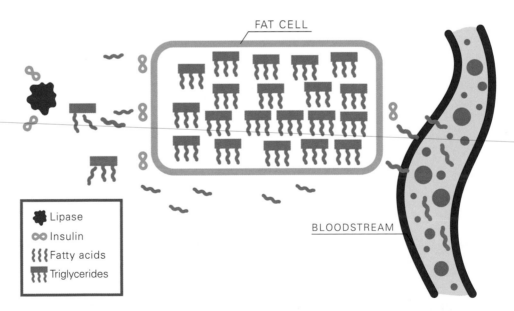

Figure 10. The new theory posits that fatty acids released outside the fat cell by the external lipase in the presence of insulin are not welcome inside because the cell is already filled with triglyceride. These fatty acids therefore enter the bloodstream. Internal lipase remains inactive, just as it normally does in the presence of insulin.

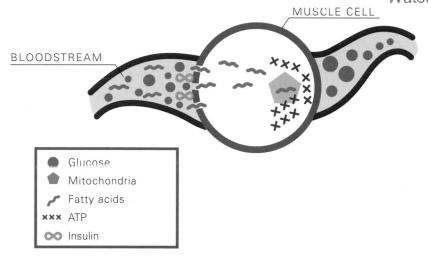

Figure 11. Muscle cells can burn glucose or fatty acids. The abundance of fatty acids in your blood triggers muscle cells to begin burning fatty acids rather than glucose. Once muscle cells have switched to burning fatty acids, even the presence of insulin cannot force glucose into the cells since they simply don't need it. As a result, glucose remains in your bloodstream, causing high blood sugar.

One irrefutable proof of my theory is that people with high blood sugar and diabetes have not just high levels of glucose in their blood, but high levels of triglycerides and fatty acids. In fact, the levels of triglycerides and fatty acids in the blood of people who overeat and are potentially prediabetic could be higher long before their blood glucose level starts a steady upward climb.[1]

If you are wondering why the body allows this switch to burning fatty acids to occur, there is actually a good reason, and it is related to self-preservation, as in many metabolic processes. In this case, when your blood glucose level starts an upward climb, the pancreas, as programmed, releases more insulin to keep the glucose level within the optimal range for your body. Insulin accomplishes this by instructing the liver to convert all the excess glucose into fatty acids and triglycerides. The body expects to be able to store this excess in its fat cells. Again, insulin helps because it energizes external lipase into action. It facilitates breaking down the triglycerides outside fat cells and triggers internal lipase to hold onto the stored fat.

[1] Kannel WB. 1985. Lipids, diabetes, and coronary heart disease: Insights from the Framingham Study. American Heart Journal 110:1100-1107

However, as your blood sugar level keeps climbing because of the lack of storage capacity, the control centers in the brain must decide whether to continue releasing more and more insulin to optimize the blood glucose level, or to tolerate a higher circulating level of glucose to preserve the functionality of the pancreas for the long-term. Part of this decision in the control centers of the brain relates to what the body can do with the high level of circulating triglycerides and fatty acids in the blood. Other than bleeding them out, which is unlikely, the only way the body has to discard triglycerides and fatty acids is through the urine after filtration by the kidneys. However, because these components are not soluble in water, the kidneys cannot remove them from the blood.

As a result, the brain opts for a balanced approach to deal with the elevated levels of glucose and fatty acids. It allows for the elevation of blood sugar, knowing that it can get rid of the glucose through the kidney and urination once the level reaches above 180mg/dl. This helps preserve the pancreatic cells in charge of secreting insulin.

As for fatty acids, the brain has two biological measures to moderate high levels of them. First, the control centers in the brain release growth hormone to instruct muscles to change their fuel preference from glucose to fatty acids. Growth hormone is produced in the pituitary gland. When we are young, it is responsible for helping us grow (hence its name). As we get older, growth hormone is released when we exercise or are under stress. It stimulates muscle to burn fatty acids at a very high rate. As you learned before, muscle cells can burn either glucose or fatty acids for fuel. They are accustomed to burning fatty acids when adrenaline is released in the body. If there is an abundance of fatty acids in the blood, your muscles will start to burn fatty acids for fuel instead of glucose. With the exception of brain cells and red blood cells, all cells in the body can use fatty acids for energy.

The second measure to facilitate the switch to burning fatty acids is executed in the liver. When fatty acid levels in the blood are high, the liver degrades large amounts of fatty acids into smaller molecules called *acetyl coenzyme A*. Just as fat molecules are similar to crude oil, acetyl coenzyme A is the ultimate refined product that every cell in the body can use in place of glucose to produce energy.[2]

---

[2] A curious example of this metabolic process happens in the Inuit Eskimo people, who can live for long periods of time on a diet that provides approximately 50% of their calories from fat. Not only can their

When the liver produces acetyl coenzyme A, it sends the molecules, packaged as small fatty acids, out into the bloodstream, which rapidly transports them throughout the body. These small fatty acids do not need a hormone like insulin outside cell walls to facilitate their entry inside. They can instantly enter cells because their fatty acid ancestry gives them a free pass through the cell membrane, which is also made of fatty acids. (Note: Although fatty acids can freely enter through cell membranes, they have to be escorted by a carrier called carnitine to enter the mitochondria for degradation to release ATP.)

Inside muscle cells, the acetyl coenzyme A molecules are released from the small fatty acids and burned to produce energy. As a result, muscles need less glucose for energy production and therefore accept less of it from the blood. Unlike the liver and the pancreas whose cells have mechanisms to escort glucose molecules in or out, muscle cells have to use all the glucose molecules that enter inside because they have no mechanism to send them out. The authority of the brain to switch the fuel inside muscle cells from glucose to fatty acids is similar to the priority that the laws of the US federal government have over those of each state. Thus, a rise in blood sugar under these conditions should be considered a normal metabolic response.

In addition, the role cortisol plays is an important side story to the balancing act being performed by the body of a diabetic in response to elevated levels of glucose and fatty acids. Cortisol, also known as the stress hormone, is released during stress. Cortisol promotes the release of fatty acids from fat. In addition, cortisol enhances the burning of fatty acids because it can get inside cells by wriggling through cell membranes. The bodies of starving people begin burning the fat stored in their fat cells. This is the best evidence of this ability of cortisol to promote fatty acid usage.

Proteins you eat are absorbed as amino acids after digestion in the intestine. Amino acids in excess of immediate use are converted into glucose by the liver. This natural capability of the liver to produce glucose from amino acids is an important tool for the body to supply fuel to the brain during a period of prolonged starvation. The difference is that during starvation, the degradation of muscle

---

livers produce glucose from the amino acids in meat, but also extensive amounts of acetyl coenzyme A, which can be burned for fuel in their cells. Thus, nature has protected the Inuit Eskimos who have little carbohydrate available to them in their diet.

proteins is the source of amino acids instead of proteins in the food you eat. In a person with diabetes, cortisol stimulates the liver to produce more glucose from amino acids that come from the overconsumption of proteins. But since the liver has no more room for glycogen, as is often the case in people with high blood sugar, it is forced to release glucose regardless of the blood sugar level or the presence of insulin.

Is the Switch Permanent?

This is not to say that muscle cells permanently switch to burning fatty acids rather than glucose. They burn whatever is most immediately available, but when your blood contains high levels of fatty acids that slip through the cell walls without difficulty, they become the fuel most often utilized. In fact, muscle cells can utilize large amounts of fatty acids to produce energy.

What's important to keep in mind about this alternate explanation of the cause of Type 2 diabetes is that too much fat is stored in your body. The fat flows through your blood and around your cells. Since your fat cells are full, they are unable to accept more fatty acids, which then circulate in the bloodstream and become the fuel of choice for your muscles. As we will soon discuss, this suggests that avoiding filling up your fat cells and emptying those that are currently full can prevent or reverse Type 2 diabetes.

Begin Tracking Your Blood Triglyceride Counts

There is an important medical conclusion we can draw from this explanation of how high blood sugar occurs. If you have not been diagnosed with diabetes but are concerned about your risk, ask your doctor to begin tracking your blood triglyceride levels. If you are overeating and your fat cells are filling up, the triglycerides your liver produces from the carbohydrate and fat in your food cannot be stored. Triglycerides cannot be excreted in your urine and therefore remain in your body.

A rise in your triglycerides over time suggests you are at risk for prediabetes or diabetes. Your triglyceride count should remain below 150 mg/dl if you want to stay below the risk level for high blood sugar. Ask your doctor to review your blood triglyceride count over the past years of blood tests and continue to track it in the future. If you detect a rising pattern, lose weight as soon as possible to begin lowering the fat in your blood and preventing the switch in fuels from occurring.

KEY POINTS

- The theory of insufficient insulin production is better explained by recognizing that each person's pancreas is working at capacity to produce enough insulin. It is the high levels of glucose in the blood from overconsumption that make it appear the pancreas cannot keep up.

- The theory of insulin resistance is better explained by realizing that in people who have filled up their genetically determined amount of fat cells, overconsumption of food causes both glucose and fatty acids to build up in the blood. As a result, their cells begin burning fatty acids rather than glucose.

- There is no defect in the ability of your cells to respond to insulin; rather, they don't need glucose at that time by virtue of already having sufficient fuel inside. If cells are doing fine without needing glucose for fuel, they have no need to respond to the presence of insulin and glucose outside the cell.

Since reading EAT CHEW LIVE, I've cut my insulin intake in half. I would normally visit my doctor every three months, and now I only need to see him every six months. I used to check my blood sugar twice a day, and now I only check it once. This book has made me a different person.

Jeanne, Type 2 Diabetic, Oregon

CHAPTER 6

The "Fatty Acid Burn Theory" Explains Many Inconsistencies

Medical scientists have long been unable to explain many anomalies about Type 2 diabetes using the insulin resistance theory. My alternative theory, the "fatty acid burn theory," resolves the following anomalies:

Why don't all obese people develop diabetes?

Why doesn't every obese person develop Type 2 diabetes if being overweight is purportedly a causative factor in insulin resistance? The fact that only some obese people develop Type 2 diabetes suggests that some other scientific explanation is needed. The fatty acid burn theory accounts for the answer.

I said earlier that your genes play a big role in your body's ability to store fat, and thus in determining when you might become prediabetic or diabetic. Some people inherit fat cells with a larger capacity for storing fat. These cells take longer to become filled with fat. Other people may have lots of stem cells that can convert to full-grown fat cells on demand. The ability of these fat cells to absorb great amounts of fatty acids explains why even some very obese individuals can maintain normal blood glucose levels. Their fat cells can store more fat and their body continues burning glucose for fuel rather than switching to fatty acids.

Why do lean people get Type 2 diabetes?

We may equally wonder why lean people can develop Type 2 diabetes. If insulin resistance is largely correlated with being overweight, why would someone who has only a little body fat become a Type 2 diabetic?

The answer is that some people may be born with small capacity fat cells. By comparison to a person with a large body structure and many fat cells, a lean person's fat cells fill up quickly with fat, initiating the fuel switch mechanism that causes their muscle cells to reject glucose in favor of burning the fatty acids freely flowing in their bloodstream. Those with lean ancestors may have inherited fewer fat stem cells. As they gain weight, the rate of conversion of stem cells to fat cells may not occur quickly enough to keep up with the amount of fat being formed. It is also possible that some people did not receive adequate nutrition in the womb and as a result have a negligible number of cells that were programmed to become fat stem cells.

Why do some women develop diabetes during pregnancy?

Diabetes during pregnancy, called gestational diabetes, has long perplexed medical scientists as it often occurs in women who have no history of diabetes, no family history of diabetes, and no weight problems or other risk factors. These women suddenly develop diabetes during their pregnancy. Soon after delivery, their blood sugar returns to normal.

Specialists in hormonal diseases often tell obstetricians that gestational diabetes is caused by temporary insulin resistance. Without proof, obstetricians are led to believe that the placenta releases pregnancy hormones and agents that interfere with the translation of instructions from the inside part of the insulin receptor on cell walls after insulin binds to its outside part on the wall. By an extraordinary coincidence, without any specific tests other than showing an elevated blood sugar level, the culprit organs turn out to be exactly the same three—fat cells, muscle cells and the liver—as those involved in insulin resistance in the general population with Type 2 diabetes.

As a medical practitioner, I always wondered why diabetes specialists insisted that both obstetricians and internists accept the insulin resistance theory in good faith just because it is presented as the cause of gestational diabetes in their textbooks. Obstetricians are required to base their decisions on how to manage gestational diabetes on this theory. This idea of insulin resistance occurring during pregnancy seems very odd to me, especially given that the great hormonal changes in a woman's body during pregnancy do not create other complications as serious as diabetes.

A better explanation for the onset of gestational diabetes is the accumulation of fat faster than our fat cells can accommodate. This makes sense given that most (though not all) pregnant women consume food in excess of their normal intake and may temporarily fill up their genetically-determined number of fat cells. In addition, it seems possible that cortisol released during pregnancy promotes the release of fatty acids from the fat cells of the mother, as well as enhancing fatty acid utilization and stimulating glucose production in the liver. The result is, of course, high levels of sugar in the blood, leading to gestational diabetes. This explanation for gestational diabetes helps explain why it appears to occur randomly, often in women who have never had high blood sugar or a history of diabetes.

Why are some children younger than 18 developing Type 2 diabetes?

Without any supporting evidence other than high levels of glucose and insulin in the blood, it is often stated that some children develop Type 2 diabetes because of insulin resistance. There is no explanation why insulin resistance would develop at such a young age or why the three organs involved are the same as in adult-onset Type 2 diabetes. The increasing incidence of Type 2 diabetes seen in people under age 18 can perhaps be best understood using the fatty acid burn theory.

In childhood and youth, the body is trying to expand its fat cell supply. Stem cells are being instructed to become fat cells. Many children become obese between the ages of 9 and 15. If the demand for increased storage is not met in a timely fashion, excess fat and fatty acids will stay in the bloodstream. Muscles will start burning fatty acids for energy while the excess amounts of glucose will elevate blood sugar, leading to the development of Type 2 diabetes in children and teens.

Why do statin medicines that lower cholesterol tend to cause diabetes?

Statins are a class of medication often used to lower cholesterol. Statin use has been associated with an increased risk of Type 2 diabetes, especially in post-menopausal women, as reported after analysis of results among women participating in the Women's Health Initiative.[1]

How are the two metabolisms—cholesterol and glucose—connected? Statins produce their effect by inhibiting the manufacture of cholesterol molecules from fatty acids in the liver. This means that fatty acids which otherwise would have been used for cholesterol formation have to be dealt with by the body in other ways. One way is that the liver uses these fatty acids to produce triglycerides, which are transported to fat cells where they are stored. This is not a problem for those people whose fat cells have the storage capacity.

However, if the fat cells are already filled, the liver stops producing triglycerides. The excess fatty acids not used for cholesterol formation remain in the bloodstream, as there is no storage for them. Once again, this facilitates the muscles switching to burning fatty acids for fuel, neglecting the available glucose and causing elevation of blood sugar and a subsequent diagnosis of Type 2 diabetes.

How exactly do our genes cause Type 2 diabetes?

It is often stated that diabetes is genetic, because insulin resistance is passed from one generation to the next. But again, there is no proof of this. The mechanism that links genetic obesity and insulin resistance in cells has not been identified. No defective genes have been found that link the two together.

In addition, there is no information to explain why lean individuals who develop Type 2 diabetes during adulthood (supposedly due to insulin resistance) would not exhibit symptoms of this condition at a younger age, since we cannot say their gene(s) were triggered by weight gain which is commonly stated to cause the production of proteins responsible for insulin resistance.

My fatty acid burn theory gives a far better explanation for why diabetes is genetic. It has nothing to do with insulin resistance, but rather with how your

---

[1] Statin use and risk of diabetes mellitus in postmenopausal women in the Women's Health Initiative. Arch Intern Med 2012 Jan 23;172(2):144-52

genetic inheritance dictates your ability to store fat and how quickly your fat cells fill up. Your genes may have given you large fat cells that fill up slowly, thus avoiding or delaying diabetes forever or at least for decades. Or your genes may have endowed you with very few fat cells, so they fill up quickly, causing your muscles to switch to burning fatty acids from your bloodstream rather than glucose. Your genes thus dictate, without your knowing, if and when you might develop high blood sugar.

This view of the role of genes in Type 2 diabetes helps us better understand who gets diabetes and who doesn't in a family. Although all humans have similar genes, genes that are active within each cell are different from person to person. Consider two siblings in a family where one parent is heavyset and diabetic and the other lean and not diabetic. Each parent contributes one-half of each pair of genes in every cell in the offspring's body. Which gene of each pair becomes active depends on many factors during the development of the fetus.

In one sibling, for instance, genes inherited from the heavyset parent could produce more fat cells and/or larger fat cells that can store more fat. This sibling could have a greater capacity to store fat and become heavier than the other sibling. The glucose and fatty acid levels in the blood could appear normal because they are stored in the fat cells. This sibling might never develop Type 2 diabetes.

The other sibling, however, despite being considered lean based on a standardized weight table, could develop Type 2 diabetes because she has genes that produced limited fat storage capacity. This sibling could fill up all her fat cells by the time she is 35 or 40, triggering the switch from glucose to fatty acid burn in muscle cells.

From this perspective, we might logically conclude that inherited genes do play a role in determining who develops Type 2 diabetes. But the difference in my theory and the standard theory of diabetes is that genetics does not cause insulin resistance. Type 2 diabetes is a function of the body's genetically-determined capability to store fat. How fast and how early in life one's potential fat storage capacity is used up varies by individual.

Another factor of genetics that could play a role as a direct cause of diabetes is our attitude and behaviors around eating. We know that our genes play a role in determining our ability to cope with stress and emotional difficulties. People who become diabetic may have a genetic predisposition to become easily stressed out. Through genetics and family upbringing, they may deal with stress by eating, even when not hungry. Our reactions to stress and our eating habits are often a function of our personality, which is influenced by our genes. We will be discussing the issue of stress and changing your eating behaviors later in the book.

Why does Type 2 diabetes sometimes disappear after weight loss?

My alternate explanation makes more sense than crediting it to insulin resistance suddenly disappearing due to weight loss. When you lose weight, your fat cells get rid of their stores of triglycerides. The empty fat cells can now accept new triglycerides made by the liver from glucose and fatty acids absorbed after a meal. Muscles can go back to using glucose more often for energy because fewer fatty acids are circulating in the blood since they are being stored inside fat cells. Blood sugar can be maintained within a normal range.

KEY POINT

- The fatty acid burn theory explains many anomalies about diabetes that have yet to be explained using the insulin resistance theory, including why all obese people do not develop diabetes, why even lean people can develop diabetes, why pregnant women get gestational diabetes, why children can develop diabetes, how statin medicines for lowering cholesterol can cause diabetes, and why losing weight can often reverse diabetes.

CHAPTER 7

No Such Condition as Cholesterol Resistance

As an interesting side trip to demonstrate the logic of my theory about the cause of diabetes, consider this comparison between high blood sugar and high cholesterol. Although the total amounts of cholesterol can be different based on one's genetic inheritance, people with high cholesterol are not viewed as having a form of metabolic resistance, so why are they when they have high blood sugar? As you will see, this analogy helps clarify that insulin resistance is an incorrect theory.

Read the following comparison between cholesterol and glucose that shows how parallel the two nutrients are.

This comparison shows that the body's metabolism handles the two nutrients in a parallel way. This is additional proof that high blood sugar is not due to insulin resistance. Let me put it succinctly: If an elevated blood cholesterol level is considered a symptom of too much cholesterol intake and/or production of cholesterol relative to need, then by extension, the elevation of the blood sugar level should also be considered a symptom of excess glucose intake relative to its use and storage in the body.

CHOLESTEROL	GLUCOSE
A molecule of fat	A molecule of carbohydrate
Absorbed from the intestine	Absorbed from the intestine
Bile acids help absorption	Sodium ions help absorption
Comes from animal sources	Comes from plant sources
Liver can make it from fatty acids	Liver can make it from amino acids
Liver releases it into the blood	Liver releases it into the blood
High blood level inhibits production	High blood level inhibits production
Transported through the cell wall	Transported through the cell wall
LDL helps passage through the wall	Insulin helps passage through the wall
Transporter guides interior travel	Transporter guides interior travel
Helps cell membrane construction	Helps cell energy production
Each cell regulates entry to inside	Each cell regulates entry to inside
Cells need less in old age	Cells need less in old age
Less intake means less in blood	Less intake means less in blood
More intake means more in blood	More intake means more in blood
Excess attaches to random sites	Excess attaches to random sites

KEY POINTS

- Cholesterol and glucose are very similar in how they are obtained from food (or manufactured in the body in some cases).

- Cells stopping their intake of cholesterol are not considered resistant to cholesterol usage.

- Similarly, when cells stop their intake of glucose, this is not due to insulin resistance.

CHAPTER 8

Why Do Diabetes Medications Seem to Work if Insulin Resistance is Not the Cause?

The first answer to this question is that much is still unknown about how many medications impact the organs. Pharmaceutical companies perform years of tests, but the approval of medications for sale does not mean that chemists and scientists understand how a specific drug impacts an organ. For example, in the case of insulin resistance in cells, there is still no specific test that proves how such resistance happens.

For this reason, drug companies have had to take many approaches to developing drugs that help people "control" their blood sugar. Note that the word "control" is the only word that can be used for diabetes because no drug has been created to "cure" the condition. But even the notion of control does not refer to mitigating the overall condition of Type 2 diabetes, but only to keeping blood sugar closer to the normal range. However, controlling blood sugar through medications without losing weight or changing your eating habits is of questionable value, as it undermines the assessment of long-term disease management.[1]

---

[1] Insulin's ability to lengthen the life span and improve the quality of life of patients with diabetes is clearly established. However, this conclusion is primarily based on the results of treating patients with Type 1 diabetes who suffer progressive damage to insulin-producing cells in the pancreas. The conclusion is less applicable to taking insulin for Type 2 diabetes.

Take fever, the common marker of an infection in the body. We can determine the effectiveness of a medication in controlling an infection by measuring changes in a patient's fever. A person with a 102 degree fever is doing worse than a person with a 99.9 degree fever in terms of how their body is dealing with the infection.

But we can also lower a fever using antipyretic agents, such as aspirin and acetaminophen. This means that measuring the temperature of someone who is taking antipyretic agents is actually an unreliable marker for determining if the infection is under control. For the same reason, we should not rely solely on measuring the glucose level in the blood as a marker of whether insulin resistance is under control. When the glucose level is lowered by a medication, a test will not reveal what is happening inside a patient's cells when it comes to insulin resistance or glucose utilization.

This lack of precise knowledge is why so many prediabetic and Type 2 diabetes patients end up frequently changing medications as they live with their condition. The medications lower the person's blood sugar, but doctors have no way of determining if the effects of the diabetes are being controlled in any meaningful way. As a result, doctors often switch medications because each drug uses a different pathway to control the patient's blood sugar.

Some diabetic medications (biguanide) are supposed to facilitate the entry of glucose into cells in the body by increasing their "insulin sensitivity," or, phrased another way, by decreasing the "insulin resistance" of the organs. However, even the pharmaceutical companies that make these drugs have not identified the mechanisms by which this feat is accomplished. In the same way we know that aspirin lowers body temperature, we know the medications lower blood sugar, but don't know exactly how.

I have many questions about medications that increase insulin sensitivity. Is it a good thing to increase insulin sensitivity in the three types of cells responsible for diabetes—muscle, liver and fat cells? If fat cells become more insulin sensitive, won't they just store more fat? Can they store an unlimited amount? If muscle cells become more insulin sensitive, will they be able to absorb more glucose? If a person does not exercise and burn that glucose, what happens to all the glucose in the muscle cell? If the liver becomes more insulin sensitive, will it produce more triglyceride using glucose? Is it beneficial to transform glucose, which is water-soluble and can exit the body, into triglyceride that can stick to arterial walls and potentially obstruct the person's flow of blood? We also don't know if it is healthy for all other organs in the body to become more sensitive to insulin under the influence of medications.

Other medications (sulfonylurea, DPP-4 inhibitor) control blood sugar by forcing the pancreas to release more insulin into the bloodstream. However, this still may not negate the fatty acid burn theory; in fact, it actually reinforces my point as to why insulin resistance is an inaccurate theory. Recall that I stated that what most medical science has interpreted as insulin resistance is simply the fact that, in a high blood sugar patient, the pancreas is producing all the insulin it naturally can but the person is consuming too much glucose. Therefore, forcing the pancreas to produce more insulin through medication is not the solution to insulin resistance at all—it's just turning the tap on more to keep up with the person's consumption of glucose-producing foods. It may temporarily help stop the patient's body from switching to using fatty acids instead of glucose for metabolic fuel. But it may also cause more harm than good. It may lead to an early exhaustion of the pancreatic cells that produce and secrete insulin, creating an early need for insulin injections. In addition, it may encourage patients to continue the same lifestyle of eating the wrong foods and overconsuming, thinking their diabetes is now "under control."

Still other medications (thiazolidinedione) accomplish the objective of lowering the blood sugar by inducing faster formation of new fat cells to create a larger storage area. These drugs do not provide direct support for the insulin resistance theory, since they have nothing to do with altering insulin production or insulin sensitivity. In fact, they actually support my fatty acid burn theory because they work by increasing storage for fatty acids, allowing cells to switch back to burning glucose. But such medications have been proven to work only temporarily, because eventually the patient's newly formed fat cells also fill to capacity. Once this happens, it has been proven that these medications stop being effective in lowering blood sugar levels.

There are also some medications (acarbose) that prevent the digestion of carbohydrates in the intestine or that (SGLT2 inhibitor) speed up the elimination of glucose, which is water soluble, through the kidneys. These drugs do not negate the fatty acid burn theory, nor do they support the insulin resistance theory.

These types of medications have many troubling side effects, such as indigestion or increasing the excretion of water through the kidney, which can lead to dehydration. It would be healthier for a prediabetic to eat less carbohydrate and produce less glucose than to risk those side effects.

In short, medications, as currently used to keep blood sugar lower, do not prove the presence of insulin resistance in Type 2 diabetes, nor do they negate the fatty acid burn theory.

Why It's Better to Avoid Diabetes Medications

If you are not yet taking medication for prediabetes, your best option is to read the rest of this book and begin implementing the recommendations so that you can remain off medications. If you are taking a medication that supposedly helps you with insulin resistance, you may be able to stop taking it as you implement the advice in this book. (I will provide recommendations in Chapter 31 for how to decide whether and when to go off your medications, working in conjunction with your physician. Do not stop taking your medications at this time; read this entire book and then discuss your situation with your doctor.)

The first reason I suggest that you avoid medications for blood sugar management is that they target the wrong problem. As this book has shown, insulin resistance is not a causative factor in high blood sugar. It is the amount of fat stored in your fat cells and remaining in your bloodstream that triggers your cells to burn fatty acids rather than glucose.

In addition, although the US Food and Drug Administration (FDA) approves medications based on extensive testing and statistical proof that the desired outcome can be achieved, almost all medications pose risks. (Whenever you watch advertisements for medications on TV, you hear warnings about such risks and have probably read the risks listed on the labels that come with your medications). It is difficult for doctors to assess dosing for almost all new medications. Some patients will need a larger dose than the recommended amount, while others turn out to need less. It may take your doctor months of trial and error to find the optimal dose.

Worse, many medications create undesirable side effects, even at the dosage considered optimal for you. To alleviate side effects, researchers often recommend a complimentary compound that can increase the efficiency of the primary medication so you can lower its dosage or a compound to reduce the severity or number of side effects. For example, taking bran, which blocks the absorption of cholesterol in the body from the intestine, to accompany a cholesterol-lowering medication can allow many patients to use less of the medication or even none at all. Unfortunately, there is no complimentary compound available to help those diabetics who are gaining weight to lower their dosage of insulin.

The use of medications to overcome insulin resistance does not guarantee that diabetic complications won't develop. Remember Sam, who was profiled earlier in this book? He suffered complications of diabetes despite using medications to maintain his A1C level below 7.

Medical Management through Fear

The real tragedy of using medications to control prediabetes and Type 2 diabetes is that it creates fear. Patients are given the scary news that they have an incurable condition called insulin resistance, a diagnosis that is presented as if it is clearly understood by experts who, in reality, have difficulty proving it scientifically. People who are considered normal weight based on weight tables are especially vulnerable to feeling fearful and confused because they are told their only recourse to controlling their blood sugar levels is to take medication. For many such people, taking medication leads to the formation of more fat—and eventually to weight gain—because their medicine-induced higher insulin production causes their liver to convert more glucose to triglycerides in the effort to keep their blood sugar in check.

The fear of having this mystery disease is often compounded by the fear of complications such as damaged eyesight, impotence, kidney failure, amputation of one or both legs, stroke, heart attack and death, all of which occur even in patients treated intensively by specialists in hormonal disease.

Some people with severe diabetes also fear its corollary problem, *hypoglycemia*—when blood sugar goes too low, causing many serious symptoms. This fear often compels them to eat even when they are not hungry, or to eat more than they need to because their medical caregiver told them to do so.

Many medical practitioners use fear to encourage diabetic patients to check their blood glucose level daily at home. Their idea is that the more you know about your blood sugar level, the better you can control it. However, there are no studies showing that regularly checking your blood sugar level results in better long-term maintenance of the blood sugar levels, a lower incidence of hypoglycemia, or fewer complications of Type 2 diabetes.

I am opposed to most medications to control blood sugar in prediabetics and in those people in the early stages of Type 2 diabetes with no other complications. My view is that medical treatment for Type 2 diabetes should be based on achieving the most significant beneficial outcomes, such as the reduced risk of having problems related to the heart, eye, kidney and other organs, and not on any supposed evidence that blood sugar values have declined. I propose these primary objectives of any therapy for diabetes:

1. Emptying out fat cells so that excess glucose can be transferred into them after conversion to triglyceride by the liver.
2. Reducing the accumulation of fat in the blood circulation to prevent the blockage of blood vessels that result in damage to the heart and brain.
3. Protecting the integrity of tiny blood vessels in the eye, kidney and feet so that they do not suffer damage.
4. Avoiding or using only on a short-term basis any medication that can produce hypoglycemia, induce the sensation of hunger, increase blood fat, or lead to significant weight gain.

In the end, the insulin resistance theory and the many fears surrounding it prevent the majority of prediabetics and early stage Type 2 diabetics from reducing or halting their dosage of diabetic medications even after losing weight and achieving lower blood sugar levels, because of the notion that they must keep "insulin resistance" under control. If insulin resistance is a scientific misconception, as I have shown you, you are missing out on the most highly effective and easiest ways to accomplish the above goals.

KEY POINTS

- Diabetic medications target the symptom (lowering blood sugar) rather than the true cause of the illness.

- It is best to avoid most medications as they are trying to treat the wrong problem—insulin resistance—and carry many risks to your long-term health.

- Medications that lower the blood sugar level make patients complacent about losing weight and making efforts to change their eating habits and avoid overeating.

If you are on diabetes medications, do not stop taking them until you have read this entire book and are implementing the recommendations in Parts 2, 3, and 4. Discuss your situation with your physician before adjusting your medications.

After implementing what Dr. Poothullil recommends in this book, I lost several pounds of weight. That was enough for me to stop the medication I was taking to lower my blood sugar. My blood pressure has also reduced to a level where I can start reducing the medication I take to control it.

Daniel, Prediabetic, Missouri

CHAPTER 9

The Politics of Maintaining the Insulin Resistance Theory

I'm excited to propose a new theory about the real cause of diabetes, as it could save many lives and help millions of people avoid diabetes and perhaps even reverse an existing condition. If people begin to accept the notion that insulin resistance does not exist, at least not as it is currently presented and interpreted as the primary cause of Type 2 diabetes, it will completely change the way that this deadly condition is treated. When people begin to understand that high blood sugar leading to diabetes is caused by overconsumption of food and filling the body's fat cells, triggering the switch in muscle cells from burning glucose to burning fatty acids, it will open up new perspectives about how we can test for prediabetes and catch the precursors of it much earlier.

The theory of insulin resistance was first published in 1931 by Dr. Wilhelm Falta in Vienna as a possible underlying cause of Type 2 diabetes. Since then, very little has been learned about insulin resistance. After over 80 years of research, our knowledge of what might cause insulin resistance in a patient with Type 2 diabetes comes down to one statement: *a change in the ratio of polyunsaturated to saturated fatty acids in cell membranes of a target organ such as muscle appears to change insulin sensitivity.* This is all that medical science has been able to prove about insulin resistance. Nothing is known about why this change would occur, why it would become a lifelong situation, or what genes may be involved in creating the faulty situation.

In comparison, consider what we have learned about human immunodeficiency virus (HIV) in just 30 years. This deadly disease first appeared in a patient in the United States in 1981. Within only three decades, HIV's structure, genome and target cells as well as its mode of multiplication and transmission have all been defined. Why have medical researchers learned so much about HIV and yet almost nothing about insulin resistance in Type 2 diabetes?

The survival of the concept of insulin resistance all these years could be interpreted as a sign of its strength and validity. However, I would argue that this concept has persisted because it has not been rigorously challenged.

Instead, by relying on one unproven explanation for diabetes, scientists have paid minimal attention to other possible explanations and channeled resources, research, and medical management in just one direction. This creates a type of self-referential circularity. Experts become comfortable supporting other experts with similar opinions, especially those based on large-scale studies that are interpreted to justify a single line of thinking. Duplicate studies to confirm or refute the results of the original study, a standard practice before using the results of one study to make treatment decisions, are often deemed too expensive or not needed because a majority of experts already think a certain way.

The unfortunate truth is that there are well-established stakeholders invested in maintaining the insulin resistance theory. They have succeeded in making sure that high blood sugar has greater name recognition and newsworthiness relative to other nutrients in the blood. Type 2 diabetes has spawned many powerful, well-funded organizations that promote this explanation about diabetes—and only this one. They organize meetings, produce leaflets, distribute magazines, help publish books, create audiovisual materials, publish treatment guidelines, provide certified educators to make patients understand the complexity of their condition and accept the permanency of it, and instruct family members and friends to make sure that patients accept this single explanation.

These organizations serve the public in many ways, such as educating people about the dangers of Type 2 diabetes. But are they doing so responsibly if they are not considering other explanations or questioning treatment objectives based primarily on improvements in a patient's laboratory values? Over time, such organizations become more interested in protecting their turf than striving for better patient outcomes. They engage professional fundraisers, even though these fundraisers keep a large percentage of the money they raise for diabetes organizations. Expenses for travel and accommodation are provided to those who persuasively articulate the mission of the organization to reassure an audience of patients and concerned family members. Money is used to promote public events and special appearances by selected celebrities who have achieved "control" of their blood sugar using medications.

Funds are raised from an appreciative public by presenting the achievements of athletes who have diabetes. However, most of these athletes have Type 1 diabetes because this population is younger and more athletic than the mostly mature adults that constitute Type 2 diabetes patients.

Any challenge to long-held positions, however scientifically pertinent it may be, can be effectively sidelined by issuing a "position paper" penned by experts demanding more research. Drug and device manufacturers, through third party groups, can pay honorariums to professionals who become members of expert panels, advisory boards, and speakers' bureaus. This also helps them gather intelligence to identify specific targets for new products. In return, the professionals are given the opportunity to endorse drugs and devices not because they improve patient outcomes, but based on factors such as reduction in blood sugar values in the case of drugs and ease of blood sugar measurement in the case of devices.

In short, the claim of insulin resistance and the management of Type 2 diabetes based on that concept will persist for the foreseeable future unless it is exposed as unscientific. In this book, I've set out to expose the truth, like the child in "The Emperor's New Clothes" who cries out, "but the emperor has no clothes on."

I am reluctant to discuss the politics of diabetes in such a cynical way, but we must begin recognizing that big corporations are influencing our healthcare decisions because they want to preserve their profits. Pharmaceutical companies have vested interests in keeping the insulin resistance theory alive because their drugs are aimed at improving insulin sensitivity, increasing insulin production, or supplying patients with insulin injections. These companies make billions of dollars on their medications and are not inclined to fund research that challenges the insulin resistance theory. Other companies benefit from the production and sale of meters for measuring blood glucose at home.

Meanwhile, the numbers of Americans with diabetes is rising to pandemic proportions. It is predicted that one in three Americans will be overweight or obese by 2050. If you learn how to control how much and what you eat and empty your fat cells by losing weight the right way, you can avoid becoming one of these statistics. Read on to find out how.

KEY POINTS

- After over 80 years of research, scientists have not been able to explain what might cause insulin resistance in a patient with Type 2 diabetes, raising doubts about the theory.

- Type 2 diabetes has spawned many powerful, well-funded organizations that promulgate this explanation about diabetes—and only this one. It is time for a new theory.

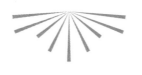

PART 2

How Your Body Takes Care of Itself

The doctor of the future will no longer treat the human frame with drugs, but rather will cure and prevent disease with nutrition.

—THOMAS EDISON

CHAPTER 10

If Children Can Do It, So Can You

You have learned that insulin resistance is not the cause of high blood sugar, prediabetes and diabetes, so let's turn our attention to how you can avoid these conditions using your body's natural mechanisms. In this second revolutionary idea about how to stop weight gain and prevent diabetes, I focus on how the brain is a natural regulatory mechanism that monitors your nutritional intake and tries to guide you towards healthy foods and proper eating habits.

I came to this conclusion by asking myself why it is that young children eat whatever and whenever they want and most tend not gain weight —at least not until they are introduced to unhealthy foods that have high carbohydrate content and added sugars and salt. Most young children have an uncanny natural ability to self-regulate what they eat. No matter how much you put on their plate, they will eat only what they need. They seldom overeat, unlike many adults who create a bloated feeling by filling their plates full, eating it all and then taking seconds and thirds.

I began to wonder if the brain is naturally programmed to eat the right amounts of nutritious food. I wondered if our cultural habits and the industrialization of food push us away from what our body intuitively knows it needs to be healthy.

In the following chapters, I will lay out my thinking about the brain as a powerful nutritional regulatory mechanism that attempts to guide you to health and survival. It literally monitors the nutrient needs of every cell in your body and tells you through your body's natural hunger and satisfaction signals when to eat, what to eat, and when to stop eating. The brain's natural ability to make the right decisions about nutrition is how babies and young children learn to eat. As we grow into adults, we too often forget what we once knew—how to listen to the authentic signals of the brain instructing us to eat only when our body needs nutrients.

KEY POINTS

- Young children have an uncanny natural ability to self-regulate what they eat.
- The brain monitors the nutritional needs of our cells and tells us when and what to eat.

CHAPTER 11

A Nutrient Primer

I have written this book to be understood by anyone, whether with or without a science background. Nevertheless, it is important that you understand some basic facts about your body in order to follow the theory and the recommendations I present. The content of the following chapters in Part 2 will make more sense to you if you have a minimal understanding of how the body works—how it digests food, how the cells function, and the nutrient composition of food. I am confident you will find this information fascinating and that it will help you appreciate your body's natural intelligence. If you are serious about losing weight, reversing your prediabetes, or avoiding diabetes, learning the basic science of nutrition will change your life.

A Primer on Your Body's Cells

Each of the external and internal parts of every active organ in your body is made up of living cells. Cells constitute the working units in the body. Cells can vary greatly in size. About 200 specific cell types have been identified in the human body.

When it forms, each cell has the potential capability of living and growing into any individual cell performing any function. As each cell is associated with and lives in an organ in the body, it becomes specialized by activating only the genes specific for the organ of which the cell is a part. For example, skin cells form a cover to protect you, nerve cells transmit and analyze information, muscle cells contract to do work, and intestinal cells allow nutrients to enter. Some cells are mobile and reach parts of the body that need help during an infection or injury. Other cells transport elements such as oxygen. Each function results in different consequences in the body.

For optimal functioning, the body needs to maintain the structural integrity of all your cells and their processes. It does this by:

- providing a comfortable environment for the cells by removing waste and excess heat,
- neutralizing any toxins in the cells,
- guiding cell growth while preventing unwanted multiplication,
- detecting and destroying invading germs,
- providing transportation for cell products that are delivered to the outside, and
- performing many other activities in a timely fashion.

Your Cells Nutrient Needs

All living cells have to carry out routine maintenance activities to survive and perform the task they are assigned. To manufacture the specialized products they need, each cell requires a specific set of raw materials, or nutrients. For example, calcium is needed for bone cells, and bone marrow needs iron and vitamins to create various blood cells. Brain cells need a continuous supply of glucose for their normal energy production, whereas muscle cells can use either glucose or fatty acids for energy, as you have learned.

Scientists do not yet know the exact number of nutrients the body needs, or whether some nutrients perform multiple functions, or whether different combinations of nutrients can accomplish the same functions as other combinations of nutrients. Since food supplies differ throughout the world, it would seem logical that the body can adapt to whatever nutrients are available to it. For example,

I mentioned that in cold climates where grains are not as readily available, the liver can manufacture glucose from animal proteins and fats.

Science has identified 118 nutrients that are used at some time for human health. No one knows with certainty how much of each of these your body actually needs or how you derive them from the foods you eat. That is why I always suggest eating a wide variety of foods to ensure you have the opportunity to ingest as many of these nutrients as possible.

118 Nutrients Your Body Uses

adenine	delphinidin	hydroxocobalamin
alanine	docosahexaenoic acid	hydroxymatairesinol
alpha-Carotene	eicosapentaenoic acid	indol-3-carbinol
alpha-Linolenic acid	epicatechin gallate	iodine
arginine	epigallocatechin gallate	iron
aromadedrin	ergocalciferol	isoleucine
ascorbic acid	eriodictyol	isorhamnetin
asparagine	fisetin	kaempferol
aspartic acid	fluoride	lariciresinol
beta-Carotene	fluorine	leucine
beta-cryptoxanthin	folic acid	linoleic acid
biotin	folinic acid	lipoic acid
calcium	fructose	lutein
carnitine	galactose	luteolin
cholecalciferol	gallocatechin gallate	lycopene
choline	gamma-Linolenic acid	lysine
chromium	genistein	magnesium
cobalt	glucose	malvidin
coenzyme Q10	glutamic acid	manganese
copper	glutamine	matairesinol
curcumin	glycine	menaquinones
cyanidin	glycitein	methionine
cyanocobalamin	hesperetin	methylcobalamin
cysteine	histidine	molybdenum
daidzein	homoeriodictyol	myricetin

naringenin	pyridoxine	sodium
niacin	pyridoxamine	sulfur
niacinamide	pyridoxal	syringaresinol
pachypodol	quercetin	tangeretin
pantothenic acid	rhamnazin	taxifolin
pelargonidin	resveratrol	thiamine
peonidin	retinal	threonine
petunidin	retinol	tocopherols
phenylalanine	riboflavin	tocotrienols
phosphorus	secoisolariciresinol	tryptophan
phylloquinone	selenium	tyrosine
pinoresinol	selenocysteine	valine
potassium	serine	zeaxanthin
proline	sesamin	zinc

Energy Nutrients vs. Essential Nutrients

Cells need energy from "energy nutrients" for their internal functions. When you are deep in sleep, your muscles are very limp. If suddenly awakened, your muscles have to be activated to get you out of bed. Without energy immediately available, muscles cannot move. There is no time to start up the energy production machinery in a muscle cell.

I discussed energy production earlier, but let's quickly review it. Energy for the metabolic activity in a cell is contained in a molecule called ATP for short (this stands for *adenosine triphosphate*). Each cell has a special area called mitochondria that prefers to use glucose to manufacture its ATP, but fatty acids can be used as well.

Here is a fascinating bit of information: Genes in the nuclei of all cells in the body come from both parents. However, the genes responsible for the mitochondria come from the mother, with rare exceptions. This means that the survival of every cell in the body and by extension the very existence of the human race is made possible by energy produced by powerhouses designed by females!

Cells are constantly manufacturing ATP, so millions of ATP molecules float around in each cell, ready to unload energy. Most ATP molecules are used up within two minutes after being made. But some remain unused, ready to be activated when your body needs energy at another time. ATP is like the batteries of a flashlight, available to power your body when you need energy.

The energy created from the decomposition of ATP may be used for whatever metabolic reaction a cell is programmed to do. For example, in some cells ATP energy is used to link amino acids together to form protein molecules. In other cells, ATP energy is used to synthesize substances your body needs such as hormones. Skeletal muscles are responsible for utilizing 80 to 90 percent of the glucose consumed to create ATP. As you can see, glucose is a vital component of the body's nutritional needs to formulate ATP to produce the energy needed for all our cellular functions, but especially muscles.

However, the continual production of ATP without a corresponding usage of it is not only a wasteful process, but also potentially dangerous. If there is too much ATP in a cell, accidental collisions between two ATP molecules can have the same devastating consequences inside the cell as two hand grenades colliding and exploding. Nature seems to have attempted to reduce this risk by a natural mechanism: when there starts to be an excess of ATP molecules, the cells slow down their usage of glucose to stop producing more ATP.

In addition to energy nutrients, there are nutrients called "essential." These are nutrients required for normal cell function that cannot be made inside the body. Essential fatty acids, essential amino acids and vitamins and minerals are categories of essential nutrients. Some, like niacin, a B vitamin, is also classified as essential because the body cannot synthesize enough of it. The human body can suffer illnesses due to the absence of essential nutrients.

What is most pertinent to our discussion of nutrients is the fact that the body can manufacture glucose using amino acids from proteins and glycerol from fats. *You do not need to eat carbohydrates, as they are not an essential nutrient in humans, as long as you are getting protein and a small amount of fat from other foods.*

The Imbalance of Nutrients in Food

Various foods do, of course, contain differing amounts of nutrients. In adults, any time essential nutrients are available only in minute quantities embedded in foods that contain a lot of energy nutrients, the body may be forced to eat an excess of the energy nutrients just to get adequate amounts of the essential ones. For instance, let's say you had a dish made of mixed nuts and only macadamias contain a micronutrient your body needs. You can't selectively pick out the macadamias. To get enough of the nutrient in the macadamias, you might have to eat five teaspoons of the mix containing all the nuts.

The result of this is that the body must sometimes store the excess energy nutrients that are not used to produce energy at the immediate time. The repeated intake of energy nutrients in excess of immediate need causes the body to increase its capability of storing energy nutrients. In short, you may be eating too much food just to be sure you are getting enough of the other nutrients from those foods. This overeating leads to fat storage, commonly known as weight gain.

Transportation of Nutrients to Your Cells

Nutrients enter the body through foods that are digested in the intestine. Following absorption from the gastrointestinal tract, most nutrients reach the liver for inspection before entering the bloodstream. This is because cells in the body can use some nutrients only after having changes made to their chemical composition by the liver.

Inside the body, nutrients are transported from one point to another using the liquid medium of blood. Blood flows through 60,000 miles of tubes called arteries and veins at a rate of 100ml per second. With the blood in the circulation travelling the entire circuit of arteries and veins on an average of once a minute, a nutrient entering the blood can reach any cell in the body very quickly. Tiny tubes called capillaries connect the arteries and veins to each other. The capillary walls are very thin and have numerous minute openings through which water and small nutrient molecules move in and out. The nutrients leave the blood and enter the fluid medium around each cell. Once a nutrient enters the fluid environment, it is available to cells within seconds. This fluid environment constantly feeds nutrients into the cells and removes waste products and puts them back into the circulating blood. Cells acquire nutrients such as glucose, amino acids, fatty acids, cholesterol, minerals, and vitamins from this fluid environment. This internal fluid contains all the nutrients needed by the cells in the body (figure 12).

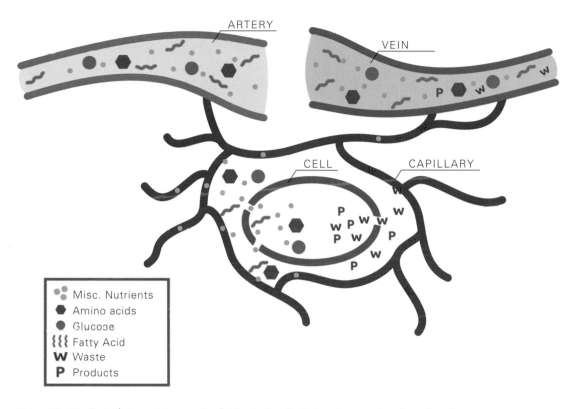

Figure 12. Capillaries bring nutrients to the fluid outside cells. Nutrients can go into the cell while waste and cell products exit as needed.

Within each cell, molecules are moved from the point of entry or from their site of production (if the cell makes other molecules from raw materials) to the area of their usage via "protein modules" that travel on thin strings of solid tracks, unlike the liquid-based transportation that takes place between organs. This method of movement is similar to transporting goods in trucks travelling on highways. Movement of these protein module transporters is powered by the ATP energy we discussed earlier, produced inside the cell from glucose or fatty acids.

How Cells Let in Nutrients

Your blood is carrying all the nutrients from digestion, but each cell needs only certain types of nutrients as the raw materials it uses to manufacture the molecules needed to fulfill its tasks. As a result, each cell has a process to select the material it will allow in and another process to control the quantity that enters.

The wall of each cell is a membrane that seals the cell completely from the rest of the body. To let in the raw materials it needs, cell walls are permeable, meaning they let molecules pass in and out. Which molecules are allowed inside a cell differ depending on the type and specialization of the cell.

On each cell wall are proteins called receptors capable of identifying signaling agents such as insulin and the raw materials needed inside. Only the right molecules can fit into each cell's receptor proteins due to their complementary shapes, which allow access while unwanted materials are denied. If this process were not in place, then the wrong materials could get inside or escape outside when a channel intended for the right material is opened. The design of this mechanism is similar to the game babies play teaching them to put the square peg in the square hole and the triangle peg into the triangle hole.

When nutrients regularly used inside the cell are present in the fluid outside, the cell assesses whether it has a need for them. If it does, the cell opens a channel in the cell wall for the nutrient to enter (figure 13). If a channel does not open, the nutrient cannot get into the cell. In other words, the presence of a nutrient outside a cell does not mean the cell has to let it in. Otherwise, cells would not have any control over what comes inside, which could disrupt a cell's internal workings.

The Body as a Cycle of Activity

The above descriptions about the cellular structure of the human body, the meaning and use of the scores of nutrients you derive from eating food, how your cells use those nutrients and how cells function to allow in nutrients show that the human body is nothing short of an enormous non-stop biological factory that has evolved to survive through an efficiently tuned pattern.

This pattern continues throughout our life unless the body is attacked by deadly germs that destroy the system's functioning, or our cells malfunction due to some other internal problem or injury. If nothing goes wrong, our biological factory runs smoothly year after year. As we age, the function of some of our cells begins to change. The walls of skin cells lose elasticity, or muscle cells atrophy from lack of use. At some point, some of our cells reach the end of their natural capabilities and we die as one or more of our organs stops functioning.

However, if you treat your body properly, respecting its cellular structures and their nutrient needs, you can live a healthy life without diseases like diabetes until you are well into your 90s or even over 100.

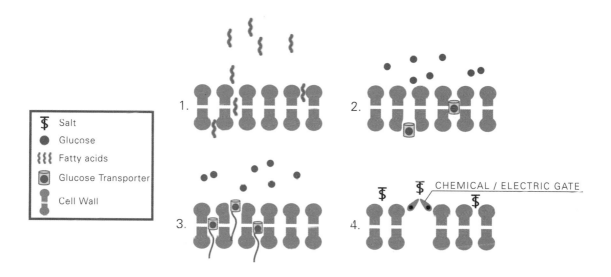

Figure 13. In general, there are 4 ways materials can pass through the cell wall.

1. Random: In the natural state, every molecule is in constant motion. If molecules in the fluid around cells get into gaps in the cell wall, they can easily enter the cell. Fatty acids gain entry this way.

2. Random-facilitated: Molecules that fit into a transporter that is already in the cell membrane can be fast-tracked to the interior. The entry of glucose into an active muscle cell is an example.

3. Reserved: In the cell wall, at the site of attachment of strings used as highways inside, there are docking facilities for specific transporters. Transporters released from inside the cells in response to the presence of insulin use these facilities to greatly increase glucose entry into cells.

4. Restricted: There are entryways in the cell wall protected by chemical agents and/or electric gates. Sodium ions use entryways protected by both to initiate muscle contraction.

KEY POINTS

- Each cell requires a specific set of raw materials, or nutrients, to perform its unique functions.

- Cells need "energy nutrients" to produce ATP to power their internal functions. Cells also need "essential nutrients"—nutrients that cannot be made inside the body—for normal cell functions. There is no essential carbohydrate nutrient.

- It is best to eat a wide variety of foods to ensure you have the opportunity to capture as many of these nutrients as possible.

CHAPTER 12

How the Brain's Nutrient Regulatory System May Work

The human body is a complex organism that survives on its intake of nutrients for energy and the manufacture of various substances the body needs. This includes the raw materials to maintain cells and grow new ones, to produce proteins and hormones, and to support metabolic processes. Unless you have taken high-level biology courses, you probably never think about your food as breaking down into literally billions of small molecules that provide the energy and essential nutrients to your cells.

If we accept the fact that the human body operates at this extremely small micro-level, where the intake of food becomes molecules that feed our cells, then we have to imagine that there is some type of regulatory system in charge of this entire operation. The body cannot be an enormous bio-chemical factory that operates chaotically without a central command to guide it and make decisions for its survival. A simple proof of this lies in the fact that we all know when we are hungry, the sensation generated by the command structure set up in the brain to inform us that we are missing nutrients our cells need to function and survive.

The point is obvious: your brain is the command center of your nutrition. The human body has thousands of control mechanisms, starting with the genes inside each cell, within each organ, at strategic locations in specific systems, and others that regulate interrelations between the organs. Similarly, the body has multiple monitoring stations reporting to centers in the brain on the levels of nutrients detected by cells, organs, locations or compartments. As such, *your brain is in direct or indirect communication with every cell in your body. It knows what those cells need to survive.*

The fact that the brain is connected to every part in your body can be proven in numerous ways. If you touch a hot stove with your finger, the brain knows which finger and sends signals to move it instantly. If you get a skin rash, your brain senses precisely where it is located and lets you know where to scratch. Your brain alerts you to an object coming close to your eyes. It quickens your breathing and heart rate to increase oxygen intake when you exercise. It wakes you up from sleep when it senses your toes are cold. When you're thirsty, it tells you how much liquid you need to quench your thirst, which is a function of resupplying your cells with water.

Each of these brain decisions is made through a background of continuous signals travelling between the cells of your body and the neurons of the brain. As those neurons function to make decisions, they are sending and receiving millions of signals from other parts of the brain, the body, and your surroundings. They are also programmed to consider stored memory. Using all the signals and memory data, they decide if you are hungry, what foods you might need to resupply the missing nutrients, and when you have eaten enough to keep your cells functioning.

The brain is the most sophisticated computer imaginable. It is composed of 85 billion nerve cells and differs from every other organ in the body by maintaining its own ecosystem. Because the brain is the command and control center for all organs in the body, it is better preserved and protected, just like a king.

One difference between the brain and other organs is that it is encased in its own "unibody" membrane, distinct from all other cell membranes in the body. Since the architecture of a nerve cell with its angular extensions, knobby projections and a tail makes it almost impossible to protect using the soft, pliable, individualized membrane that protects other cells in the body, nature has designed a special membrane enveloping the whole brain and spinal cord as if they were a single cell. This envelope, called the *meninges*, has three layers. The tough outer layer lines the bones that make up the skull and spine. The middle layer contains blood vessels and connecting filaments. The inner layer adheres firmly to the surface of the brain and spinal cord and is pierced by tiny blood vessels that bring nutrients to the fluid around cells in the brain and spinal cord.

The fluid around the brain is also different from that in the rest of the body. The concentration of glucose in the fluid around the brain is 30 percent less than the fluid around other cells in the body. In addition, unlike the fluid around other cells, which comes from tiny blood vessels, the fluid around the brain comes only from designated areas. This prevents unneeded molecules and harmful agents such as bacteria that may be traveling in the bloodstream from entering the brain fluid.

The idea that the brain can keep track of your nutrient needs at the cellular level throughout your body is completely in alignment with every other activity that the brain monitors and regulates. The brain keeps track of millions of sensations in your body every day. It stores millions of pieces of data that compose the knowledge you have accrued throughout your life. It records and organizes tens of thousands of individual memories—your first day at school, your first kiss, the swimming pool where you learned to swim, that little café in Paris you fell in love with, and thousands more. Your brain's language center recalls the hundreds of phonetic sounds you need to speak one or more languages. All of this processing takes place through electro-chemical activity that goes on inside your brain cells.

When it comes to regulating your body's nutritional needs, your brain is no different in its extraordinary capabilities. Science does not know for sure where such nutritional computing might take place in the brain, but it is possible that there are brain neurons that are constantly updated on the inventory of nutrients in your body. Starting at birth, your brain is probably tracking all the nutrients you eat. Meanwhile, the various organs and their cells seem to detect the nutrients circulating around them and can determine when the stock of raw materials necessary to their functions is running low.

The two systems running together form a tight feedback loop. The body informs the brain what nutrients it needs and the brain directs what your body needs to eat. The brain does this through a variety of mechanisms, starting with the generation of the sensation of hunger, which, if ignored, intensifies into a growling stomach, to a sensation of fatigue and low energy, to a powerful desire making you crave food.

In most cases, the brain's signal is a straightforward message of hunger, telling you to consume foods that contain a variety of energy and essential nutrients that your cells commonly need on a daily basis. On occasion, the brain sends a message that you are deficient in one or several specific nutrients.

If you don't believe this, let me ask you a question: Did you ever crave something badly, and once you ate or drank it, had a clear sensation that your body got what it needed? For instance, have you ever craved orange juice, bananas, or red meat? Could your craving mean that your body desperately needed Vitamin C, potassium, or iron—and your brain knew it? It's evident that food cravings are not random messages from the brain but rather an alarm telling you your cells need a specific nutrient.

The brain's "nutritional regulatory system" is no different than other regulatory systems the brain maintains. The brain tracks and regulates the manufacture and delivery of hormones to cells throughout your body precisely when they need them. It also tracks and regulates the level of red and white cells in the circulatory system. The brain is the CEO of our nutritional regulatory system in the same way it is the CEO of every other bodily system that keeps you alive.

KEY POINTS

- Your brain is in communication, either directly or indirectly, with every cell in your body and knows what those cells need to survive.

- The brain's "nutritional regulatory system" is no different than other regulatory systems the brain maintains, such as your hormonal system that responds to your immediate needs.

CHAPTER 13

How Your Brain Tracks Nutrients

What is the nature of the mechanism that the brain uses to identify nutrients in food? How does the mechanism work to track the nutrients entering the body? How does it track when nutrients are depleted in the body and more are needed? This is all vital information the brain must have to determine when you should be hungry and when you should be full. Once again, the answer points to a very sophisticated system of nutrient detection and communication between the brain and the various parts of your body involved with food intake and nutrient distribution. This chapter will explain this mechanism in detail.

The Brain's Nutrient Sensing System

Fingerprints are unique to each individual, with each person having a distinctly different pattern of waves and lines on their digits. A computer can match an incoming print with one in its stored database and identify an individual with 100 percent accuracy.

The brain is no different when it comes to recognizing nutrients. Every nutrient has unique physical characteristics that allow the brain to identify it, based on signals received from receptors designed for nutrients. This means that even a single nutrient molecule could generate signals to the brain when it fits into its receptor.

The capability of reacting to molecules in the external environment is called *chemical sensing*. All living things possess the ability to recognize chemical molecules. Within a short time after encountering any set of chemical molecules, we have to decide whether to tolerate or avoid them. This reliance on chemical sensing allows us to detect nutrient-rich foods and avoid harmful substances.

Our sensations of smell and taste generated by the brain are based on chemical sensing. You can recognize the fragrance of a perfume or the smell of gasoline within seconds of encountering it. The same goes for food. As you walk through a farmer's market, your nose picks up the scents of fresh vegetables and herbs. Your brain knows the difference between smelling peaches and basil, strawberries and lavender. If you pass by a restaurant grilling meat and a bakery next door baking fresh bread, you can smell the odors and immediately distinguish between the beef and the bread.

Your smell receptors likewise respond to the physical properties of the molecules in the food you put in your mouth. Your smell receptors can immediately determine if there is garlic in the pasta on your fork or Swiss cheese on the bite of sandwich you just took. Your sense of smell is one mechanism by which your brain knows what food is around and what you are about to eat. If you have never smelled an odor before, your brain attempts to correlate it with something it knows and make a judgment about what nutrients might be in it (figure 14).

In addition, the receptors on the tips of the taste cells in your mouth are exposed to incoming nutrients in food and react to molecules before you consume them and again as you chew. The stimulation of the various taste receptors generates electrical signals via the movement of ions such as sodium through their membrane. The receptors are in almost continuous communication with the brain through these signal transmissions. The rate of signal transmission from these cells increases proportionally to the strength of nutrient stimulation. Your mouth senses if the tomato sauce is watery or bursting with Italian tomato flavor, or if the hamburger is unseasoned meat or loaded with mustard, garlic, salt, and pepper.

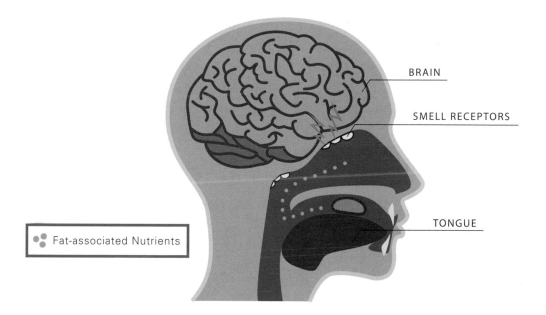

Figure 14. Your smell receptors utilize chemical sensing to identify nutrients in your mouth and send electrical signals to your brain to appreciate what you are chewing.

As the brain processes incoming signals from the taste sensors, it analyzes the chemical nature of the molecules. It searches the brain's memory banks and recognizes them as being pleasant (or not) and having one of the following characteristics: sweet, sour, salty, savory, or bitter. Your brain tells your mouth to keep chewing to savor the flavors or to spit the mouthful out. If your brain does not recognize the molecules, it attempts to make a comparison to other foods you have eaten in the past in an effort to decide whether you want to keep chewing or reject the food.

In this way, as you eat, food is crushed to a pulp inside your mouth, mixed with other foods you would not mix on a plate on the table, diluted with water, wine, alcohol or other assorted liquids, mostly warmed but sometimes cooled and tossed around the tongue. This allows your brain to extract the assortment of signals coming from a seemingly chaotic mix so it can make a decision about taking the next bite. This mechanism in the brain is no different than the way it can distinguish individual sounds coming from an automobile, an animal, a child, and a radio—even when they all occur simultaneously—and still decide on a course of action.

In short, the brain has a powerful capacity to evaluate and combine signals triggered by different nutrients in your smell sensors and taste receptors into a completely meaningful experience. This interpretation is also combined with emotions stored in your memory from previous encounters with the same food to create the pleasure or distaste you have from this experience of eating.

How the Brain Knows Your Current Nutrient Status

Your brain must ensure that all needed nutrients for all cells in the body are present in the fluid medium surrounding each cell. One way the brain might acquire this information is by monitoring the level of nutrient in a sample of fluid that flows around cells. This measurement can then be compared against the availability of each nutrient from areas in the body where it is stored. The brain can then determine which nutrients are low, to what degree they are lacking and, as a consequence, which nutrients must be replenished as soon as possible.

So where does the brain get the information about the nutrient content of fluids around the cells of your body? The location: *in your mouth*. The signaling mechanism: *your taste buds.*

As just discussed, taste buds detect nutrients entering the mouth and pass that information to the brain. One proof of how sensitive the capability of taste receptors is can be seen in how quickly you know the composition of many foods as soon as they are in your mouth. If you introduce just a few milligrams of a nutrient such as salt, sugar, cinnamon, vinegar, or anything else into your mouth, your brain knows about it instantly. This means taste cells have an established transmission pathway in touch with the brain in real time.

If the concentration of a nutrient is low in the fluid around the living cells of your body, it is also low in the fluid around the taste cells. Receptors capable of monitoring nutrients are already present on taste cells. They have a direct transmission pathway to the brain through the nerves that serve them. As the concentration of different nutrients becomes low, messages are sent to the brain (figure 15). The brain also receives information from organs such as the liver and fat cells as to the availability of nutrients already in storage. In addition, brain cells themselves can detect the level of nutrients such as glucose molecules in the fluid around them. Smell receptors can function in a similar fashion because, although located in the roof of the nasal cavity, they are extensions of brain cells.

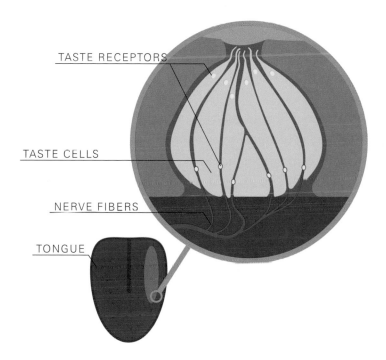

Figure 15. Receptors on the base of your taste cells are connected to nerves that provide the brain with information about the nutrient content of the fluid around it. The brain uses this information along with information from other parts of the body to determine what nutrients the body may need, and produce the sensation of hunger when the total nutrient need reaches a threshold level.

Saliva secreted by glands located in the oral cavity can be another source for analysis by taste receptors. In addition, as the saliva passes down the throat and crosses the path of air from the lungs coming forward, volatile elements can be picked up and presented to the smell receptors. This is similar to sensing the food just consumed when you burp with your mouth closed.

Using all these signals, the brain assesses if a threshold has been reached and there is a need to replenish one or more nutrient(s) in the body. The brain then sends your conscious mind a signal—this is the first hunger sensation, telling you it's time to eat. At the same time, the brain sends signals to the liver and other storage areas to release nutrients so that critical levels can be maintained in the blood. The release of stored nutrients such as glucose from the liver moderates our hunger intensity for a while, suggesting this mechanism evolved because we need time to find food. Eventually, if you don't eat soon enough, the brain has a second warning system that reminds you again to eat. This mechanism works through the release of hormones that alert you more forcefully using real physical signals, such as hunger pangs in your stomach walls and a rumbling of fluids therein.

The brain's nutritional regulatory system also monitors the water level of the body. Receptors in the mouth constantly check for water molecules. If they become significantly reduced, the receptors generate signals to the brain that the body needs more water. These signals are augmented by others sent from the internal organs indicating they are lacking in fluids. For example, cells in a specialized part of the kidney are constantly exposed to water and continuously monitor water molecules. They inform the brain about the state of hydration in the body. The brain cells themselves may also sense the amount of water molecules in the fluid around them. From these combined signals, the brain can decide when to generate the sensation of thirst.

Located at the point of entry of food into the body, your taste and smell receptors are uniquely positioned to serve as executors of this natural, elegant and simple regulatory system. It is the same system that prompts you to bend your nose to a flower after smelling just a whiff of its fragrance or walking towards the oven when you smell apple pie. It is the same system that makes a hungry newborn avidly reach for the mother's nipple after getting a taste of the breast milk. It is the brain's intelligent monitoring system that prompts a toddler to ask specifically for milk to drink one time and water the next when both beverages are available and the toddler is thirsty. It is the same system that prompts adults to suddenly "feel like" eating steak, fish, or eggs or to crave orange juice, though by the time we become adults, many other factors, such as our culture, taste preferences, and psychology also play a role in determining what we want to eat or drink, often overriding what our brain tries to tell us about our cellular nutritional needs.

The beauty of this system is that the hardware needed to establish a fully functioning regulatory mechanism is already in place by the time each human is born. The first four or five years of life are devoted to making connections between nerves, testing the workings of nerve cell groups, and establishing cause and effect relationships between the sensation of hunger and the nutritional impact of eating. Through the repetition of the same feeding actions over and over, nerve connections become established, associations between tastes and nutrients are made, pathways for the travel of signals from taste buds and smell receptors to the nerve cells become solidified and the relationship between the intake of different foods and the brain's ability to assess their nutrient composition become established.

What Triggers the Hunger Signal?

The brain's regulatory system uses cellular fluids as an indicator of the nutrients missing from the body. This system informs the brain of the constantly shifting nutrient inventory in a matter of seconds and triggers our hunger signals.

However, nothing about human biology is simple, so it is probably true that the cause of the hunger sensation may be based not on just a single missing nutrient, but rather on a complex formula the brain must take into account. With the human body needing close to 100 different nutrients in order to be healthy, the level of any specific nutrient might be relatively low at any given time. If a deficiency in just one nutrient caused the hunger sensation, then we would conceivably walk around getting hunger signals all day long. It is more likely that the signal for hunger is based on the accumulation of signals about the deficiency of multiple nutrients. Only when the combined signal strength reaches a threshold level does the brain finally generate the sensation of hunger.

Imagine the performance of an orchestra of stringed instruments, wind instruments, drums and cymbals. Each instrument contributes its share of different sounds to create beautiful passages of power and strength. Hearing one instrument play its part alone could never give you the same sensation of melody, harmony, rhythm and tone as hearing the entire orchestra.

This is very likely similar to how the brain accumulates signals about nutrient deficiencies. The brain may receive lots of signals that slowly blend together to create a powerful enough impetus that the brain is prompted to sound the alarm, "Time to get food."

KEY POINTS

- Every nutrient has unique physical characteristics that allow the brain to identify it, using chemical sensing.

- The brain can identify incoming nutrients and internal nutrients in the fluid surrounding the cells from signals generated by taste and smell receptors, as well as other internal monitors.

- The brain generates the sensation of hunger when the accumulation of deficiency signals about multiple nutrients reaches a threshold level.

CHAPTER 14

An Experiment that Proves the Brain's Capacity to Regulate Nutritional Intake

Is there any proof that your brain knows you need specific nutrients and directs you to eat them? Is there any evidence to suggest that humans have a sophisticated mechanism to select from among various natural foods and consume enough quantities to meet the nutrient needs of a growing, active and changing body?

The answer is yes. The evidence comes from a highly controlled and validated experiment that took place over 70 years ago using infants who were newly weaned from breast milk and given a wide selection of foods to choose from on their own, without any adult prompting or assistance. In this experiment, it was demonstrated that infants would naturally choose an assortment of foods that provided all the nutrients their bodies needed to remain healthy and growing.

While we might be tempted to think that infants would choose the same food over and over, or might veer towards only sweet or salty foods, or might not eat enough or too much, this experiment showed that *babies' food choices and taste preferences are driven by their nutrient needs.* The experiment seems to verify that the brain has a mechanism to monitor the nutrient levels in the body, assess what new ones are required, and stop food intake as nutritional needs are met.

Summary of the Experiment

Between World Wars I and II, Dr. Clara Davis conducted an experiment with 15 infants, age six to eleven months. None of the babies had been given foods other than formula or milk before the study. This age was chosen because the children had no experience of adult foods and no preconceived prejudices or biases about them. The children remained in the program for six months to six years.

Four infants were underweight, suggesting that they had not been getting adequate nutrition. Five had rickets, a medical condition due to inadequate intake of nutrients such as vitamin D and/or calcium.

The children were presented with a selection of 34 different foods of both animal and vegetable origin. These items were known to contain all the necessary nutrients such as proteins, fats, carbohydrates, vitamins and minerals that humans need for survival. The items were selected because they could generally be procured fresh year round. They included only the following:

Water; grade A raw milk and cultured milk; table salt; uncooked apples, bananas, orange sections or strained orange juice; fresh pineapple either finely cut or ground; finely cut, peeled peaches; finely cut, peeled tomatoes; beets, turnips, cauliflower, lettuce and spinach cut or ground; baked potatoes and bananas; cooked apples, carrots, peas, and cabbage cut or ground. Oatmeal (steel cut) and wheat (whole wheat ground and not heat-treated) were served raw. Oatmeal, corn meal (yellow) and barley (whole grains) were cooked in a double boiler for three hours. To prepare the grains, one cup of cereal was cooked in five cups of water. Ry-Krisp made of whole rye flour and water with one percent common salt added was offered. The meats were lean beef and loin lamb chop from which 50 percent of the fat was removed before grinding and broiling without water loss. Cooked bone marrow was also offered, as was bone jelly made by boiling five pounds of veal bones in three quarts of water until one quart remained. Chicken, sweet breads, brains, liver and kidneys were finely cut and cooked in covered casseroles in a steamer. Fish (haddock) finely cut or ground, cooked in a covered casserole in a steamer was also offered, as were eggs served raw and soft poached.

All foods were prepared as simply as possible, unmixed and unaltered except in some cases by cooking in the simplest manner. Some foods were served both raw and cooked. Cooking was done without the loss of soluble substances and without the addition of salt or seasonings. Each food, including salt, milk and water was served in a separate dish on a tray.

The infants were free to eat with their fingers or in any way they could. If an infant consumed an entire portion of an item, the size of the portion was increased at the next feeding to ensure that when some was left, it signified that the infant had eaten all he or she wanted of it.

The infants were seated in chairs at a low table. All foods were placed in front of the infants on a regular tray without any order in their arrangement. The tray was placed on the low table. Two teaspoons were provided, one for the infant to try to use when it wished, the other for the nurse who sat beside the child. The nurse did not offer food directly or by suggestion. Only when an infant chose a dish, either by reaching or pointing, did a nurse offer a spoonful and only if the infant opened its mouth for that food was the food put in. When the child had definitely finished eating, usually after 20 to 25 minutes, the foods were taken away.

During the course of the experiment, the infants had regular physical examinations, blood tests, urine analysis, and x-ray examinations. They were observed for changes in appetite, evidence of discomfort or abdominal distress after eating, vomiting, constipation or diarrhea. Stools were examined for undigested food.

The study found that no infant failed to manage their own diet. All of them maintained good appetites. The infants often greeted the arrival of their trays by jumping up and down, and showed impatience while their bibs were being put on. Once placed at the table, having looked the tray over, they usually devoted themselves steadily to eating for 15 or 20 minutes. When their hunger had moderated, they ate intermittently for another five or ten minutes, playing a little with the food, trying to use the spoon and offering bits to the nurse.

None of the infants ever gave any evidence of discomfort or abdominal pain after eating or was constipated. Except in the presence of parenteral infection, there was no vomiting or diarrhea.

There was no clue as to what influenced the infants in choosing the foods they tried and whether the choice was a random one or whether they were attracted by color or odor. It was clear that after the first few meals, the foods most desired were promptly recognized and chosen. The infants reached without hesitation no matter where the desired food was located on the tray, ignoring other foods that were nearer at hand or brighter in color. Each infant in the beginning chose some foods that he or she spat out after tasting. The infant did not choose these foods again, demonstrating that even by this age, infants develop specific tastes.

Every infant ended up with a unique diet, different from every other infant. None of the diets were predominantly cereal and milk with smaller amounts of fruit, eggs, and meat—which is usually considered optimal meals for this age group. Their tastes changed unpredictably from time to time. Although they showed decided preferences, it proved impossible to predict what any infant would eat at a given meal. Even the daily consumption of milk varied from 11 to 48 ounces. They ate salt only occasionally, often sputtering, choking and/or even crying bitterly after putting it in the mouth but never spitting it out and frequently going back for more, repeating the same reactions.

One of the most striking results was that meals often consisted of strange combinations by adult standards. For example, a breakfast of orange juice and liver, a supper of eggs and milk. A tendency was seen in all the infants to eat certain foods in waves, i.e., after eating cereals, eggs, meats or fruits in small or moderate amounts for a number of days, an infant would follow that with a period of a week or longer in which a particular food or class of foods was eaten in larger and larger quantities until astonishingly large amounts were consumed. After this, the quantities would decline to the previous level.

The infants did not show any clear preference between raw and cooked foods. Attempts to mix foods or pour milk over any were not observed. Several solid foods were usually taken at each meal, and liquids—milk, orange juice, and water—were drunk at intervals during the course of the meal, as is the habit with adults.

The average daily calories consumed in the diets were found to be within the limits set by scientific nutritional standards for the infant's age and body weight, except in the few instances in which the infants who were undernourished before weaning exceeded the standard when they entered the study.

Five infants had rickets when they entered the study, reflecting a defective deposition of calcium during bone formation. Since vitamin D plays an important role in bone formation, Dr. Davis decided to put cod liver oil, a rich source of vitamin D, on the trays along with other foods. One child with rickets voluntarily drank 178 cc. of pure cod liver oil and 80 cc. of cod liver-incorporated milk in 101 days. About the time the blood calcium and phosphorus reached normal levels and bone x-rays showed the rickets to be healed, he stopped drinking these.

Regardless of their condition at the time of entry to the study, within a reasonable period, the nutrition of all infants improved based on physical examination, urinalysis, blood counts and bone x-rays. The examining pediatrician commented that they were a fine group of children from both a physical and a behavioral standpoint.

The Striking Conclusions about the Brain's Role in Our Eating Habits

While this study was conducted over 70 years ago, the results seem to confirm that humans have a natural regulatory mechanism in the brain that helps us know what we should be eating to obtain our nutritional requirements. This is a striking result in the context of today's world of overconsumption, where many have lost control of their eating habits. For example, eating a food in increasing volume for a few days and then decreasing the quantity shows the presence of a mechanism that dictates the choice and amount eaten until the immediate nutrient need is met. Taste preferences did not seem as important among the infants as some type of regulatory information telling them what foods their body needed.

Even the body's need for salt became obvious in the experiment. While the infants invariably expressed displeasure at eating raw salt, they consumed it voluntarily, even when another food with less salt and more obvious palatability, Ry-Krisp, was readily available. This suggests the presence of a mechanism to choose a food with the maximum concentration of the needed nutrient, salt, from among the items available.

It would also seem that the one infant with rickets who voluntarily partook of cod liver oil validates the presence of a sophisticated regulatory mechanism capable of monitoring nutrient levels inside the body and even identifying nutrients needed to cure a specific defect. After consuming cod liver oil the first time, the infant's choice to keep consuming it seems to show that the brain could identify the food as having the nutrient he needed, then monitor the quantity of the nutrient necessary to consume until his rickets were cured.

What possible mechanism enabled the infants in this study to make the right choices to acquire adequate amounts of needed nutrients? I submit that the clue lies in the enthusiasm exhibited by the infants upon the arrival of the food tray. This is a clear indication that the control centers of the brain are activated by pleasure sensations generated through taste and smell signals after the children became familiar with the items on the tray. These signals then trigger the selection of the right foods containing the nutrients needed at that time.

As the infants ate and their nutrient intake met their nutritional needs, the pleasure of eating subsided and the children started to slow down their consumption. If fullness of the stomach were the determining factor in terminating each meal, the quantity consumed should have been predictable and similar for each infant from one meal to the next, but this was definitely not the case. Keep this point in mind because recapturing the same anticipatory excitement of each meal and the enjoyment of each food you eat till the pleasure subsides are the keys to your life without diabetes. I will show you how to accomplish this in Chapter 30.

Applicability of the Experiment to Adults Today

If you accept that this experiment is evidence of how the brain monitors and regulates the intake of nutrients in infants, it is only logical that this regulatory mechanism also applies to adults. There is no evidence to suggest that any of our natural regulatory mechanisms in the body change as we grow into adulthood. For example, our body's mechanism to regulate our water intake through our sense of thirst does not appear to change as we grow from infancy to adulthood. Our mechanism to regulate breathing remains the same between infancy and adulthood, based on the concentration of oxygen in the blood, the need to exhale carbon dioxide, and the need to maintain proper acidity of the blood.

Thus, when the adult brain knows we are lacking in nutrients, it prompts us with the same clear message as it did when we were children: *I'm hungry, and this is what I need to eat.*

KEY POINTS

- Between World Wars I and II, Dr. Clara Davis conducted an extensive experiment with 15 infants, age six to eleven months; the results demonstrated that babies voluntarily choose their foods according to their nutrient needs.

- The experiment appears to verify that the brain has a mechanism to monitor the nutrient levels in the body, assess what nutrient(s) are required, direct you to choose a food containing the needed nutrient(s), and stop food intake as nutritional needs are met.

PART 3

Reconnecting with Your Authentic Weight

The more you eat, the less flavor.
The less you eat, the more flavor.

—CHINESE PROVERB

CHAPTER 15

Food Intake:
Need vs. Desire

In Parts 1 and 2 of this book, you learned that insulin resistance is not the cause of high blood sugar leading to prediabetes or full-blown Type 2 diabetes, but rather that filling all your fat cells causes your muscles to switch from burning glucose to burning fatty acids. You next learned that your brain monitors and tracks your nutritional needs and prompts you to eat the foods that supply the necessary nutrients for your cells.

In Part 3, we will be focusing on my third revolutionary idea that can guide you to losing weight and improve your eating behaviors. This is the concept of connecting with your "authentic weight"—the body weight at which your brain knows your body is operating on an even, healthy keel. When you become aware of your authentic weight and begin respecting it, this awareness can be a powerful driving force to encourage you to lose weight and reconnect with your body. Being motivated to achieve and stay at your authentic weight will help you change the unhealthy overeating habits that caused you to veer away from maintaining your body at its optimal weight.

I am not a proponent of diets, so my recommendations for how you rediscover your authentic weight have no basis in counting calories, purchasing prepackaged foods, or following a program of diet fads. Rather, in Part 3, I aim to teach you a new way to think about losing weight that I am sure you will find radically different from what most diet and weight books suggest. For example, I will discuss the role of exercise and why it will not help you lose weight. I will next examine the impact of several food groups that people commonly misunderstand—fats, carbohydrates, natural sugars, and salt. For the past several decades, science has identified fat as the leading cause of weight gain and diseases such as atherosclerosis and heart attacks. This myth is increasingly being debunked, and as you will learn, the real culprits in your meals are carbohydrates, sugars, sweeteners, and salt. These foods create the metabolic processes that lead you to weight gain and potential diabetes.

Obviously, there is some part of the brain that seems to convince many people to overeat and consume unhealthy foods that taste good, even though they know deep inside that these foods have little nutritional content and make them gain weight. There is, in effect, a battle happening inside the brain for control of your body's nutrition. Which part of your brain you allow to win will determine whether you stay healthy and live a long life or whether you develop high blood sugar and perhaps diabetes and its dangerous complications.

KEY POINTS

- When you become aware of your authentic weight and begin respecting it, it can be a powerful driving force to encourage you to lose weight and reconnect with your body.

- There is, in effect, a battle happening inside the brain for control of your body's nutrition. Some part of your brain knows how to eat for nutrition, while another part is swayed by other desires.

CHAPTER 16

A New Perspective about Your Weight and Its Link to Diabetes

Weight is the first topic that we need to review in launching you on a journey towards a healthier lifestyle free from high blood sugar and the fear of developing diabetes. The concept of weight is often misunderstood. This chapter aims to give you a new perspective about body weight and how much you "should" weigh, especially in the context of preventing or reversing diabetes.

Reframing the Link between Weight and Diabetes

Weight plays a key role in preventing diabetes, but it is not because of the old theory that being overweight triggers insulin resistance. As you learned, high blood sugar is not a function of your weight triggering insulin resistance, but rather a function of your fat cells filling up, causing your muscle cells to begin burning the excess fatty acids circulating in your bloodstream before they burn glucose. This is why lean people can also develop high blood sugar. They can also fill up their genetic inventory of fat cells. It is a false correlation that being overweight causes diabetes due to insulin resistance.

The subject of weight is tricky, and even many medical professionals do not understand how weight affects health. A lot of health issues appear to be caused by, or aggravated by, extra weight but are actually not. Consider a person who weighs 300 pounds and has knee joint problems. It is often assumed that the person's weight strains the knee joint and so losing weight will relieve the strain. However, there are many 300 pound people who do not have knee joint problems, while there are plenty of 150 and 180 pound people who do. Since knee pain is not specifically caused by the accumulation of fat, all we can say is that losing weight *may or may not* help someone's knee pain. This same logic applies to many health conditions that are not specifically caused by weight gain.

When athletic people who are in the process of building muscle gain weight, a false assumption can be that the weight gain will lead to prediabetes. However, muscle weighs more than fat. Someone who gains 15 pounds after strength training is not necessarily on their way to becoming prediabetic simply because they put on weight.

One of the dilemmas of assessing what a person's "normal" weight should be is that the standard weight tables used in most medical contexts are poorly calibrated. You are probably not aware that the most common weight guidelines used by doctors in the US are based on data originally obtained in 1943 from the Metropolitan Life Insurance Company, or MetLife. The tables were made because MetLife was trying to calculate the insurance risk of people dying. The company asked their policyholders to self-report their height and weight when they purchased life insurance and used that data to prepare a chart of "ideal" weights based on the lowest mortality rates among their customers. People who lived the longest were deemed to have been at the ideal weight when they filled out the survey at the age they were. However, there is no firm linkage between weight and mortality, so these weight tables are effectively useless.

In 1985, a new height and weight chart was prepared by the Gerontology Research Center, National Institute of Aging, Baltimore, MD, which attempted to calculate a healthy weight range for adults of all ages. The problem with this chart is that the range of weights for each height is very broad and cannot help predict whether someone might become prediabetic. No one has been able to pinpoint a clear "cut-off" point in any weight range that determines what extra amount of weight triggers high blood sugar.

For example, let's say you are 35 years old, stand at 5 feet, 5 inches tall and weigh 147 pounds. The height/weight chart says you are normal, as you fit inside the bracket between 115 and 149 pounds. But let's say that after developing pre-diabetes, you lose 12 pounds and your blood sugar returns to normal. How could you have known that your non-diabetic weight should have been at the lower end of the range rather than the higher?

It's Your Body Fat Ratio That Counts

If you want to prevent or reverse diabetes, a more useful guideline is not a weight/height chart but rather the ratio of your body fat to your weight. This can help predict the risk of diabetes in a person because it provides some indication of how much body fat you are carrying. One method used to measure body fat is underwater weighing. The differences in the densities of fat, muscle and bone allow an accurate determination of the percentage of body fat.

However, this method of measuring your body fat ratio doesn't indicate the location of your fat distribution, i.e., the amount of fat in each location of your body, which helps to understand the potential fullness of your fat cells. A cheaper and faster measure is the Body Mass Index (BMI), based on a mathematically derived formula that takes into account the effect of your height on your body weight. More height means more bone and muscle, which weigh more, so this measure is a little better because statistics show that people with a higher percentage of body fat tend to have a higher BMI than those who have a greater percentage of bone and muscle. You can measure your BMI at the website for the National Heart, Lung, and Blood Institute.[1]

The BMI test can be misleading though, as its formula cannot distinguish fat mass from muscle mass. Muscle weighs more than fat. This means that if you are very muscular at any height, it adds to your weight, skewing your BMI. A test might indicate that you are overweight or obese, when in fact you are not. The reading would be false if it indicated you are at risk for diabetes just because your BMI is high.

The BMI test can also underestimate body fat in older adults who have lost muscle because its formula assumes a certain amount of muscle for each height.

---

[1] See http://www.nhlbi.nih.gov/guidelines/obesity/BMI/bmicalc.htm.

If you have lost muscle due to aging or lack of exercise, you will have more of your weight stored as fat. This means your BMI might indicate that you are in the normal range when in fact you have too much fat.

Given these flaws, using the BMI test as a measure of one's risk of diabetes is problematic. Instead, some experts suggest that you can assess your risk of diabetes (as well as heart disease) by noting where you carry your fat. If you are storing most of your body fat around your waist—e.g., you have a fat belly—rather than at your hips, you are putting yourself at a higher risk. Statistics show the risk of diabetes increases in women who have a waist greater than 35 inches and in men with a waist greater than 40 inches.

"Feeling Your Authentic Weight"

I believe that every person has access to a wise method for determining if you are too heavy and carrying too much fat in your body, which sets the stage for the switch from glucose to fatty acids as the fuel your muscles burn. This method is what I call "feeling your authentic weight." Whenever I tell people about this concept, almost everyone knows exactly what I am talking about. It is intuitive and immediate—and I assume you understood it as soon as you read it in the same way that you intuitively know what someone who talks about "justice" or "equality" or "morality" means without their having to define it.

We all have a sense of our authentic weight because our brain tells us what it should be. Perhaps you have never thought about your authentic weight, but once you begin reflecting on it, you will likely get a good sense of what you should weigh.

Paying attention to your authentic weight is your brain's way of signaling that you are healthy or that you are exceeding the weight that is right for you. If you are in tune with your authentic weight, you immediately sense it when you gain a few extra pounds as you start to feel uncomfortable. Your stomach may feel bloated, you may feel some muscle pains, or you may feel slower and more tired. Exceeding your authentic weight may prompt you to become aware that you need to lose some pounds.

Unfortunately, most people tend to rationalize their weight gain once they exceed their authentic weight by a few pounds. They attribute it to stress, aging, busy days at work, family obligations, lack of time to exercise, the discovery of a new food they love, or simply to the fact that other people around them are gaining weight, too. Such rationalization becomes increasingly convincing over time because your brain tends to believe ideas it repeats.

Let me elaborate on why getting back in touch with your authentic weight is the key to knowing how much you should weigh so you can strive to reach this weight. As stated, you cannot use standardized tables of height and weight, nor can you count on your BMI to determine your weight. Your authentic body weight is a measure of the total mass of all components of your body, including bone, muscle, organs, blood, fat, and water. The role of each of these components of the body in contributing to one's weight differs in every individual in the world. You could be tall and small boned with lots of muscle, or short and big boned with regular muscle—and weigh the same. Only you can intuitively know your authentic weight based on what your brain assesses.

Your authentic weight can also change as you exercise and age, because the contributions of each component of weight can change. If you begin working out, adding muscle, you might gain muscle weight but your brain knows you are still in your authentic range because it takes into account your extra muscle mass. If you are aging and losing muscle, but gain 10 pounds in body fat, your brain will sense that your authentic weight is now skewed towards fat, even though you may weigh the same.

Are You Ready to Be Honest About Your Weight?

To avoid Type 2 diabetes, your goal must be to take back control of your body and rediscover your authentic weight. Your weight is right for you if your brain knows that your fat cells are not full and your blood is not full of fatty acids and glucose. You can also look in the mirror and see whether you are carrying layers of fat in your abdomen, hips, or buttocks. Regardless of where you land on a standard height/weight chart or BMI measurement, let your brain tell you the truth. Your health risks, particularly for diabetes, are related ultimately to how much of your weight is in your blood in the form of fat or sugar and how much of it is in your fat cells.

If you are unable to rediscover your authentic weight, you can consider the body weight you had when you were in your mid-20s as a close approximation of it, provided your blood sugar and triglyceride levels were within normal range at that time. That is the age at which you probably reached your full height and your bones reached their maximum density. Any weight gain since that age will reflect in general the increase in pounds you have added due to storing fat and/or building muscle. (For most people, as they age, weight gain is due to storing fat!)

Another way is to use all known standards to determine weight, such as the standard weight/height measurements and BMI. Shoot towards the weight recommended by these scales, but be sure your blood sugar and triglyceride values are within their normal ranges. Then, use your intuitive sense and brain messages to remain at about your personal authentic weight.

If you have difficulty feeling your authentic weight, you may be forced to rely on blood triglyceride levels to assess your health risks related to weight gain, unless the medical community can develop more sensitive markers such as an elevated fatty acid level.

KEY POINTS

- Being overweight based on a weight table does not automatically mean you are heading for high blood sugar or diabetes due to insulin resistance.

- The ratio of your body fat to your weight is a better guide to adjusting your weight, though this method also has flaws.

CHAPTER 17

So Why is It So Hard to Control Your Weight?

If full fat cells cause your body to burn fatty acids and create the conditions for high blood sugar, why did nature make it so easy to fill our cells with fat and so hard to eliminate the fat we have stored? Wouldn't it be great if you could eat a certain type of food and cleanse your body of stored fat and fatty acids in your bloodstream in one fell swoop?

Unfortunately, one of the most perplexing medical problems in the developed world today is that our food has become plentiful and our cultures have become highly food-focused. Most of us are conditioned to eat and enjoy food from the day we are born. Our eating habits are developed when we are children and reinforced as we age, so changing them as adults becomes a mental struggle against decades of ingrained behavior around food. Our eating patterns and habits become so natural, so automatic and so unchangeable that we do not even recognize them as being culturally determined or under our complete control. Evolution did not create humans who require three meals a day plus a few snacks and desserts. Our genes don't dictate that we need to eat 3-decker club sandwiches, French fries, cinnamon buns, sugary cereals, potatoes au gratin, and cupcakes to supply our bodies with nutrition.

I will be devoting several chapters to teaching you about how to eat to rediscover and maintain your authentic weight—and thereby set up new conditions for a healthy, robust metabolism that will not trigger the fatty acid burn switch and cause you to become diabetic. Let's start by briefly examining some of the reasons why millions of people cannot figure out how to lose weight and rid themselves of their fat stores.

It Begins in Childhood

During the first year of life, you triple your body weight. Your parents, grandparents, uncles, aunts and other relatives and family friends encourage your efforts, marvel at your achievement, and adore your bodily appearance. This begins your love affair with food—and with good reason, as you wouldn't survive infancy without nourishment. All the loving care and attention your parents pay to your eating habits as well as to all the other human traits you develop at this time such as smiling, talking, walking, laughing, and learning are oriented towards helping you stay alive.

After the first year of life, you actually stop gaining weight at the same rate as you did in your first year, because nature has built-in control mechanisms to match your food intake more closely to the growing needs of your body. This is the period when your cells need many thousands of nutrients to build your organs and expand your brain cells. Your eating habits are dictated by your body, not by the conditioned behaviors of the adults around you. How many two year-olds do you know who eat three meals a day just like adults?

Even at five years of age, most children do not eat according to family habits or culturally-determined behaviors. They eat what they want, when they want. If they eat excess food during one meal, they compensate for it with reduced intake during subsequent meals because their brain knows how much nourishment they need. Young children listen closely to their brain's signals telling them when they are hungry and when they are satisfied. They intuitively eat to stay at their authentic weight.

As we grow up, though, most children begin falling into patterns highly influenced by their family's eating behaviors, their taste preferences, and their culture. They have meals at the same time their parents do. They eat the food choices given to them—whether that be meat and potatoes in some families, Chinese food in others, or vegetarian in still others. Children and teens also begin to expand their taste preferences as they experiment with foods they see on TV, in advertisements, and in the movies—sugary cereals, fancy cupcakes, chocolate-covered anything, and perhaps even sushi for the very brave.

If you are an active child and teenager, you may be able to eat everything in sight—even if it is full of carbs, sugar, and fat—and still maintain your weight within a range of a few pounds. Most teens do not become prediabetic because their metabolism utilizes all the food they eat. They are lengthening bones and building muscle mass. Even if they keep some fat in storage, it is quickly used to produce energy when they need it between meals.

The problem is, however, that our eating habits are being increasingly assaulted by the modern world and the foods being manufactured for most people to eat. We see millions of children falling prey to unhealthy snack foods and meal choices that are aggressively marketed to them. These foods are full of added sugar, carbohydrates, and salt, and children and teens overconsume them without realizing they might suffer health consequences down the road. Lured by these products, children are losing their body's natural ability to remain at their authentic weight at increasingly early ages. The levels of childhood obesity are rising everywhere in the Western world.

We are now seeing prediabetes and diabetes in younger and younger children. Millions more children engage in food consumption habits that will put them at risk of being overweight, if not obese, and prone to Type 2 diabetes by the time they are young adults. This is precisely why the predictions indicate that by 2050, 1 in 3 Americans will be fully diabetic, up from 1 in 10 adults today. This statistic is shockingly high because it includes today's children who will grow into adults with eating habits that push them into diabetes.

Our Eating Habits Pursue Us into Adulthood

If you are an adult reading this book, whatever poor eating habits you developed during childhood persist into adulthood. You probably enjoy eating foods that remind you of pleasurable experiences and memories of good times from your past. It is also likely that you have adopted other unhealthy eating habits as you aged, based on other factors. You may have developed a taste for eating a lot of certain types of ethnic foods whose flavors and spices are different from what you grew up with. You may eat between meals because you are stressed out. You may eat too much at dinner time because you skipped lunch during the day and are now enjoying sitting around the table talking to your family or guests. You may have added alcohol into your meal times or between them without considering the extra calories that alcoholic beverages add to your daily intake. If you are a parent, you are teaching your children these same unhealthy eating habits.

When all these factors are combined, it is easy to see how you can lose touch with your authentic body weight and your brain's signals for hunger and satisfaction. Instead of paying attention to these signals, your other habits and behaviors take precedence in your brain. I am convinced that most people are completely aware when they are eating unhealthy foods and overeating. They can hear that voice in their brain telling them to stop eating so much, or to eat something better, because the brain has been monitoring their nutritional needs. But they ignore that voice because other voices in the brain assure them that they will derive pleasure from other foods or from continuing to eat.

I have news for you. You will not avoid prediabetes or reverse Type 2 diabetes unless you begin to listen to your brain's signals about your nutritional needs and how much to eat. You must alter your dietary habits and return to your authentic weight. For many of you, this means emptying your fat cells as much as possible, as well as taking back control of your food intake.

KEY POINTS

- Children listen closely to their brain's signals telling them when they are hungry and when they are satisfied.

- We are all being assaulted by industrial foods loaded with carbohydrates, sugars, and salts.

- As an adult, instead of paying attention to internal signals, behaviors that produce immediate pleasure take precedence in your brain.

CHAPTER 18

Exercise is Great, but not for Weight Loss

In almost every book on weight management, exercise is usually mentioned as the key to losing weight and keeping it off. On the surface, you would think this makes sense. When you exercise, your muscles send a message to the brain for additional fuel. The brain, in turn, sends a signal to the liver to release glucose not only to supply fuel to muscles, but also to brain cells. In addition, the brain sends another message to fat cells to release more fatty acids that can be burned as fuel, thus emptying them. This makes room in fat cells to once again accept triglycerides made from fatty acids. This process will then help your body transition back to burning glucose rather than fatty acids.

Many people, especially those young in age, do lose weight using exercise as a tool. However, I have a completely different view of exercise. My opinion is that it is *possible* to lose weight through exercise and, in the process, reduce your blood sugar levels and prevent or reverse prediabetes. However, it is not *probable* that you'll lose weight. Most people cannot rely on exercise as their primary method to lose weight. Before you object, let me present a variety of reasons that people seldom take into account when they begin exercising to lose weight.

First, most people simply do not exercise enough to accomplish the goal of emptying their fat cells. Exercising burns very few calories relative to one's daily intake, especially if you are already overeating. A woman weighing 140 pounds may expend 270 calories by walking 3.5 miles in one hour, 390 calories by riding a bike for one hour and going a distance of 10 to 12 miles, or 430 calories by running 30 minutes at a speed of 7.5 mph. But if she is doing one of these forms of exercise only two or three times per week, all the while consuming 1800 or 2000 calories per day, she will hardly make a dent in depleting her fat cells. The same goes for men, although the numbers are slightly different.

Add to this the fact that exercise itself usually makes people feel hungrier. You go out for a walk, a bike ride, or to the gym and you then return home and eat even more. Exercise often makes people crave sweets, or think they deserve a reward of an ice cream or a chocolate. So if your strenuous exercise regimen is accompanied by increased calorie intake, you might even end up gaining weight rather than losing it.

Another problem with exercise is that it does not have the same impact on weight loss as you age. It is very difficult to keep up the level of activity needed to maintain a negative calorie intake when you have aging muscles. What used to take 20 minutes to burn 300 calories now takes 40 minutes or even an hour since there is a gradual decrease in the ability to maintain skeletal muscle function and mass.

Some professionals encourage exercise for weight control with the reasoning that the resting metabolic rate stays elevated after stopping the exercise, which helps to spend more energy. It is true that there is a gradual decrease in the resting metabolic rate after early adulthood and you can increase it with exercise. However, as we have seen, if the amount of energy expended on the actual exercise doesn't make a significant difference in your weight, the after-effects will be even less.

What Exercise is Good For

I don't advocate exercise as a tool to lose weight because I believe exercise is neither necessary nor intended for weight management. If exercise were necessary for weight control, an overweight person who is eating and exercises should not feel hunger until his or her weight is re-optimized. Conversely, a person who is eating but not exercising should keep on gaining weight, but not everyone does. For example, every senior citizen should be gaining weight given that seniors typically slow down in their activities. If exercise were the body's natural mechanism to maintain weight, then we would all feel the urge to exercise after a sumptuous meal, just as we feel the urge to move when listening to music with a strong beat. Instead, most of us feel lethargic after a heavy meal.

Exercise is valuable for one's health, but not for weight management. Physical activity is vital to the body, starting from childhood. Children who are active at all age levels and get pleasure from it are more likely to maintain active behaviors into adulthood.

The primary objective of exercise is to condition the lungs, heart and muscles, regardless of your body weight. Conditioning develops reserve capacity available for use when you need it or when you become sick For example, an older person who does not exercise may have the capacity to deliver one liter of oxygen per minute to the tissues and a reserve capacity of three to four liters per minute. An athletically fit old person may have twice that much reserve. When an athletically fit older person develops a condition such as pneumonia, he or she has more available respiratory reserves. The same is true of a conditioned heart in an athletic older individual—it can pump more blood with less effort than an unconditioned person and has the reserves to help that person through a serious illness.

Similar reserves can be expected for the actions of other organs and systems in the body of someone who exercises. For example, conditioning allows your muscles to work longer before your brain senses the stress of exercise and makes you feel tired, compared to the brain that is not conditioned to exercising muscles. The ability of the human body to cope with unexpected events can be improved if the reserve capacities are maintained.

Additional benefits of exercise come from improved blood circulation which helps the brain to think more creatively and the skin to have a better tone. The sustained elevation of body temperature you get from exercise also improves the immune system and defense mechanisms of the body and makes it easier for the transfer of glucose from the blood into active muscle cells, as you learned earlier in the book. For many people, the addition of exercise in their daily routines also reduces stress and offers the key to greater psychological happiness and wellbeing, even if they are gaining weight.

If you are diagnosed with prediabetes or diabetes, exercise can help your muscles burn more fatty acids as well as glucose thereby reducing their levels in your blood. So please do exercise, but don't view it as your key to losing weight.

KEY POINTS

- It is possible to lose weight through exercise, but most people cannot rely on exercise as their primary method to maintain weight.

- Exercising burns very few calories relative to one's daily intake, especially if you are already overeating.

- Exercise is valuable for one's health—to condition the lungs, heart and muscles, and to improve blood circulation—but not for weight management.

CHAPTER 19

Among the Ways to Lose Weight, Only One Works the Best

If exercise is not the way to lose weight, what is? You are undoubtedly familiar with these five other techniques:

1. medication to restrict absorption of fat from the intestine,
2. medication to reduce appetite,
3. psychological intervention,
4. surgery either to remove fat (usually in the thighs and/or abdomen), or restrict food intake
5. restricting your intake of certain food groups, particularly carbohydrates, added sugars, and salt

The reality is that the first three techniques seldom work. Unfortunately, the vast majority of people who use medications or psychological intervention as currently practiced end up regaining the weight they lost within a few years. Taking medications to lose weight also carries many risks and side effects. A medication (orlistat) that inhibits the enzyme responsible for digesting fat in the intestine may cause frequent oily bowel movements. A medication (sibutramine hydrochloride monohydrate) that suppresses appetite may increase blood pressure and cause constipation and insomnia.

Meanwhile, the fourth method above, surgery, may be useful for some people, but it is costly, has its own risks, and requires a lengthy period of recuperation. Some people have come out of weight loss surgery with life-threatening and permanently harmful complications.

The Best Way to Lose Weight

By far the best way to return to your authentic weight is to focus on #5 in the list above—restricting your food intake. You need to recalibrate your relationship with food—what to eat and how much of it. The next few chapters will go into detail about the most egregious culprits that have caused you to gain pounds beyond your authentic weight— carbohydrates, added sugars, and salt.

You may feel you have heard these ideas before, but as you read the coming pages, you will see that my recommendations differ from other books and programs. Most current weight reduction programs simply do not help you understand the role your brain's regulatory mechanisms can play in naturally guiding your food consumption. If you spend time learning about the role of your food choices, you will begin to understand how to lose pounds in the most natural way so you can return to your authentic weight and permanently alter your eating habits while you enjoy eating what you want.

If you are genetically programmed to store a lot of fat in your body, it may be difficult for you to significantly reduce your body weight anyway. So for you, the only real choice you have is to adjust the quantity and type of foods you eat.

Let me emphasize one point: *it doesn't matter how fast you lose weight, as long as you do it in a way that helps you reduce blood sugar.*

Don't pressure yourself into believing you need to lose weight quickly. If you think about it, you probably gained weight slowly over many years, so there is no reason to think your body needs to lose weight any faster than you gained it. I suggest that one pound per week is sufficient and an appropriate goal. Your body will not miss one pound each week. The value of going slowly is that you can see what works best for you regarding how you change your eating habits, what side effects you might experience and how long you can sustain your new weight. What counts is having a downward trend in your weight week by week, month by month, until you arrive at your authentic weight. In addition, losing weight slowly gives your internal power-generating systems time to get used to the change in fuel usage, and it helps you maintain your skin elasticity without the danger of developing the sagging that occurs from rapid weight loss.

Overcoming Our Cultural Addictions

Our cultural environment has a negative influence on our food choices. We are living in an environment where food is cheap and plentiful. We inhabit a body that is designed to store lots of fat. Capitalist companies heavily promote cheap fast food meals that look good and appeal to our taste. We also live in a country where the medical community as a whole does not have consensus to undertake a national campaign to halt the pandemic that is prediabetes and diabetes. Given these conditions, it takes a lot of mental stamina to be vigilant about your weight and your consumption of unhealthy foods—despite having a sophisticated brain that has evolved to keep you eating nutritiously so you can survive.

I hope you will find the rest of this book an eye-opener and empowering force you can use to find your authentic body weight and maintain it for the rest of your life.

A Special Note for Women about Losing Weight

The worst way to lose weight is to focus on fixing your body image (an external motivation), rather than on getting in touch with your authentic weight (an internal motivation). This problem is especially true among women in our society. The desire for attention and acceptance by fellow humans, especially those who are considered "better" than you in appearance, is embedded in human nature. But in a society that uses the physical figure as the defining feature of female attractiveness, a media industry that promotes the feminine body appearance as the easiest way to appeal to others, and a weight loss industry constantly promoting "easily achievable" targets, too many women are fixated on controlling their body weight as a means to feel happy and confident.

The tragedy is that body appearance for women is fast becoming a generational problem. A young girl growing up today in a household with a mother who herself has failed to maintain an authentic body weight may be encouraged not to gain weight. The mother, unable to understand or unwilling to look at the reasons for her own failure, may be motivated by a desire to spare her daughter the frustration, humiliation, and feeling of helplessness that came with her own repeated attempts at weight maintenance.

The daughter, full of youthful energy and confidence, then tries to get support from her most trustworthy source, her peers, many of whom may be in the same situation. Collectively, they look for guidance at the most accessible source of information—the media, which then perpetuates stereotypical female body images without any medical science or health reasons to support claims. As these young girls grow into maturity, they tend to experience the same results as their mothers because they never learned anything meaningful about weight maintenance other than how they are supposed to look. The mothers never discussed with their daughters the important topics related to health and weight for lifelong happiness rather than external beauty and appearance.

This cycle often continues as young girls become women and start their own families. Fearful of gaining weight and aware of the difficulty of maintaining authentic body weight based not only on their own experience but that of their mothers, these women tend to repeat the pattern of focusing on external beauty with their own daughters.

I feel this is a vicious cycle that requires action by the medical community. We need more medical professionals to promote the body's natural regulatory mechanisms about food, teaching moms and daughters to recognize and respect when they are hungry and when they are satisfied. Without such guidance, we will continue to have generations of mothers who teach their daughters what they should look like based on their own failed experiences and expectations of beauty. Girls, in turn, will continue to feel pressure to disconnect from their own natural control mechanisms of food intake in favor of media and stereotyped cultural images of beautiful women who are held out as models of appearance and lifestyle—while teaching them nothing about health and longevity.

KEY POINTS

- Most people who use medications or psychological intervention end up regaining the weight they lost within a few years.

- It doesn't matter how fast you lose weight, as long as you do it in a way that helps you reduce blood sugar. One pound per week is a sufficient goal.

- The worst way to lose weight is to focus on fixing your body image. Body appearance for women is becoming a generational problem, with mothers passing on to daughters a cycle of unhappiness about their body.

I have been a diabetic for 17 years. After implementing what Dr. Poothullil described in this book, I have lost 33 pounds and reduced my insulin usage to one-fourth of what I was taking before.

Wayne, Type 2 Diabetic, Oregon

CHAPTER 20

The Myths of the Balanced Diet and Eating in Moderation

If losing weight and avoiding prediabetes depends more on your diet than on exercise, the question is, what should you eat and how much of it?

You Can't Balance Nutritional Needs

The most common rubric you will hear about eating healthy is to eat "a balanced diet." The idea of eating a balanced diet is a very complex one made up of bits and pieces of information and attitudes acquired over generations, with many of these attitudes in conflict. As currently understood, a balanced diet is based on eating a variety of foods within and among the five food groups in order to derive all the nutrients your body needs. You are advised to balance each type of food, choosing, for example, foods that are low in fat if you have already consumed something high in fat. You should also moderate your portion sizes so that you can enjoy all the foods you like while controlling the intake of calories and total amount of fat, saturated fat, cholesterol, sugars and sodium. The serving amounts are determined based on the average content of nutrients in foods and average daily utilization of the same nutrients in the body adjusted for age, gender and activity level, starting from age two years and up.

The problem with this view of a balanced diet is that the nutrient amount currently recommended for intake during each day and each meal is a calculated average based on scientific studies of the actual amounts people consume over a period of time. Although it can be helpful to have some type of recommendation based on averages from different studies, it is still a rough approximation. The actual amount of nutrients that most people consume during meals is usually vastly different.

Calculating averages is a useful research tool to understand what has already happened in the past. Averages can also be helpful when you are planning for your body's expected needs over a period of time in the future. Knowing the exact amount of a nutrient to be consumed based on a study is reassuring when it is an actual value determined by specific, measurable conditions.

However, averages are not very reliable. The accuracy of averages in research on nutrients depends on how well the study conditions are controlled, whether the study subjects have the nutrient under study in their system already, and, if so, at what level, and the concentration of the nutrient in the food consumed. In my view, applying a recommendation to any specific individual is suspect because people do not live in controlled environments.

Your nutritional requirements depend completely on your individual situation, which changes day by day. One day you may have a busy 16-hour schedule, full of activity and stress. Following that, your body may be severely deficient in certain nutrients needed to produce more stress hormones. Another day, you may do intensive physical exercise and your body becomes deficient in the minerals and vitamins used to produce energy. You have to take into account these differing circumstances in your daily life. It is almost impossible to suggest a balanced diet based on average daily use under these conditions.

Moderation is Meaningless

Researchers and commentators often proclaim that if people exercise "moderation" in eating a meal, the quantity consumed can be within 'acceptable' limits, although they seldom define the meaning of acceptable "moderation" or how to achieve it. Ironically, it has been shown that those who exercise a high level of self-control experience faster satiation of "unhealthy foods" and slower satiation of "healthy foods," compared to people with lower self-control.[1] Why would this be? One theory is that people with higher self-control pay more attention to what they eat when the food is unhealthy, and this attention leads them to feel more satiated and eat less.

Meanwhile, it is clear that getting people to agree on the definition of a "healthy food" is challenging. According to one's preference, the meaning of healthy can be based on the energy content of food, on the food group it pertains to, or on the nutrient content of the food. You will probably have difficulty getting ten people to agree on any food whether it is healthy or unhealthy.

The fact is, most people still need a clear action plan to understand eating healthy food in moderation and prevent overconsumption. Without a method, we are at the mercy of whoever is serving us the food. If you go to a restaurant, the portions designated as "small" might conform to the concept of moderation. But without a precise agreement as to what quantity constitutes the meaning of small, every restaurant can and does differ in the size of its portions. In addition, restaurants can simply rename their portion sizes (and change prices) to make customers believe they are eating moderately. Worse yet, many restaurants simply change the appearance of their servings to make unhealthy food look like a healthy version of it, or they re-label old recipes with a healthy name to fool customers into thinking they are consuming good food.

When it comes to eating in moderation based on the energy content of the food, it is well accepted that satiation during a meal has little to do with the caloric content. Knowing the energy content of the portion served seldom helps people eat in moderation. Just go to any fast food restaurant and you will see people consuming 1500 calories in one burger meal. Yet, they may believe they ate in moderation and still feel hungry.

As a result of such confusion, this book advocates listening to your brain to guide you in determining the quantity consumed during a meal, because the quantity of needed nutrients changes from person to person and from meal to meal based on internal and external conditions. I advocate connecting to your

---

[1] Redden JP, Haws, KL. February 2013. Healthy Satiation: The Role of Decreasing Desire in Effective Self-Control. Journal of Consumer Research. Vol. 39

authentic weight and paying attention to how well your brain informs you, if you listen to it, about how much to eat. That's why the recommendations in this book are revolutionary and different.

Variability is the Real Key

The concept of eating a balanced diet is different in this book. There are no specific foods that I believe constitute a requirement for the body. The variety of foods available in different parts of the world attests to the fact that humans can eat whatever is available in their local area and derive all the nutrients they need.

Instead, my emphasis is on eating a wide variety of foods to ensure that you are getting all the nutrients, such as glucose, amino acids, fatty acids, vitamins and minerals that your body needs for growth, energy production, repair and maintenance. Each cell in the body requires multiple nutrients to survive, sustain internal functions and create products such as enzymes, hormones and proteins. It is not the presence of a single nutrient that produces the unique biological effect of a cell, but a specific mix of nutrients in the fluid around each cell and the readiness of the cell to respond. What is thus needed is a diet that changes with the nutrient needs of the body.

So if you have a tendency to eat the same foods over and over, branch out and try new fruits, vegetables, spices, and meats. Vary your menu using the most seasonally available, freshest items because fresh foods that are eaten in season still contain most of their nutrients. Try new recipes where ingredients are mixed differently to create various combinations of nutrients in the food you consume. Think of eating as a chance to explore the great diversity of nutrients available to humankind.

KEY POINTS

- Eating a balanced diet is based on a calculated average using scientific studies, but what constitutes a balanced diet is only an approximation. Eating in "moderation" is a vague, seldom defined recommendation.

- Portion sizes can be deceiving in restaurants, and calorie counts have nothing to do with feeling satiated after eating.

- Eat a variety of foods to ensure you maximize your chances of eating all the nutrients your body needs.

I've had Type 2 diabetes for 25 years and have been on an insulin regimen for years. I've been doing what EAT CHEW LIVE says for the past month and I've already cut my insulin down to one-third of what I usually take. This book has made a big difference in my life.

Martha, Type 2 Diabetic, Oregon

CHAPTER 21

Things You Need to Know About Fat

Because losing fat from your fat cells is the first thing you must do to lose weight and get on the path to a healthy lifestyle free from the threat of diabetes, the first topic we will discuss is *fat*.

Fat is the body's preferred method for storing energy nutrients that are not put to immediate use. As I explained earlier, full fat cells trigger the conditions for high blood sugar and diabetes. The question is: Why does the body store fat? Why do people become overweight, and suffer related health complications? Why doesn't the body naturally find ways to eliminate fat if it leads to so many problems that get in the way of long-term survival? The answers to these questions offer interesting insights into how you can lose weight and prevent diabetes.

The Old Theory of Why We Store Fat

You have probably heard it suggested that our evolutionary ancestors developed the capacity to store energy in the form of fat because they faced periods of famine. The genes responsible for creating fat cells to store energy were a survival advantage and were passed on from generation to generation. If you have ever tried to lose weight, only to rebuild fat after a few months, the theory claims it is those same genes that are responsible for replenishing your fat stores. Although food has become plentiful year round, these same genes continue to make it possible for people to store large amounts of body fat and become overweight or obese.

If the above theory is correct, then these genes should be present in all modern-day humans. But if this were true, it leaves these questions unanswered.

- If storing fat is beneficial for survival, why would nature evolve to allow fat to clog our blood vessels and cause us to die (unless, perhaps, the consequences of starvation are worse)?
- If the theory is valid, then why don't most of us start storing fat and become obese when we are children, since these genes are present in the body at birth?
- Why don't obese people have a survival advantage with all their stored fat?
- Why haven't lean people disappeared from earth if their genes don't allow the hoarding of food?

Given these questions, is storing fat truly a survival advantage? Because the body cannot survive on stored fat alone, the theory is suspect. The body also needs some proportional amount of stored protein, carbohydrate, vitamins, minerals, and trace elements, but these elements don't have storage locations in the body.

One might argue that the body needs a modicum of fat in storage at least to generate enough energy so we can go out and find our next meal. For this purpose, however, we would need only several pounds of fat because each pound of stored fat packs 3500 calories, enough energy to last a few days. If your body had 2, 3, or 5 pounds of fat, that would be sufficient. But millions of people carry 10, 30, 50, and even 100 extra pounds of fat. Did their genes allow them to gain all this weight just for survival storage?

The human body needs water. It's very likely that our human ancestors faced periods of drought, just as they faced periods of famine. But there is no evidence suggesting humans have developed the capacity to store water to survive periods of drought. So why would human nature have evolved to help us store fat, but not water?

The Real Reason We Store Fat

If there is no evolutionary proof that we store fat to survive, what might be the reason? I propose that the reason we store fat is because it is the best way humans have to ensure that we have immediate access to all the nutrients our body needs. Our short-term nutritional needs, and not our long-term survival, is the reason. Let me walk you through this rationale.

Let's start at the newborn period. The human body is designed to accommodate gains in both weight and height from birth. In the first four months of life, an infant drinks breast milk or milk-based formula containing about 61,000 calories and doubles their body weight. On average, an infant uses up to a third of the energy contained in lactose for growth and some for maintenance. But this leaves some sugar that needs to be stored.

This could explain why, at the age of four months, fat tissue already accounts for almost 50 percent of an infant's body weight.[1] After this period of rapid infant growth is over, fat tissue accounts for a smaller percentage of body weight at age one and an even smaller percentage at ages two and three. But during this period of rapid growth, the infant consumes nutrients at a rate faster than at any other time of life. So why do infants store fat?

An infant's body is like the construction site at a housing development. After demarcating and clearing the land, streets are laid, utilities are buried, sites are marked, materials are brought to each site, houses are built, appliances are installed and power, water and sewer lines are connected to each house. All these can be done on a programmed timeline, with supplies coming in at just the right

---

[1] By the way, if you are still skeptical about my theory that insulin resistance is not a causative factor in type 2 diabetes, consider this. Medical textbooks state that obesity creates the conditions for the inherited genetic propensity to develop insulin resistance to occur. According to the American Council on Exercise, obesity is defined as having body fat over 25% for men and over 32% for women. Based on these criteria, almost every baby is obese from their newborn period to about age one since about 50% of their body weight is fat. Yet, babies develop neither insulin resistance nor type 2 diabetes, even those who develop it as adults. It is illogical to think that insulin resistance is a result of excess body fat.

time. If there are delays or interference, the timeline can be changed and the inconveniences tolerated.

In an infant's body, however, there can be no delays in supplying nutrients. The construction of many organs progresses at the same time as the functional capability of every organ increases. Cells are multiplying by the millions and each cell is manufacturing proteins by the thousands after erecting assembly lines within. Messages are sent and received through chemical, molecular, or electrical signals; nerve lines are established for instant communication between sites; vascular tubes are laid for transportation routes and nutrients are brought to the site by the liquid conveyer system, blood.

Because all this growth occurs simultaneously, a wide variety of nutrients have to be available on a 'just-in-time' basis and in sufficient quantities. Their absence could produce significant delays in construction, with consequences that could be damaging for life. For example, if nutrients needed to produce proteins are not available, construction of cells and their assembly lines may not be completed. If proteins needed to produce hormones are not available, organs may not be activated in a timely fashion. Any significant interruption of the construction or activation of an infant's organs could diminish their quality of life correspondingly. We know that nutritional deficiencies account for many diseases in children, from deficiencies in teeth to bone growth to defects in organs.

Even if the necessary nutrients become available after a delay, restarting the construction may not be possible. This is because when the original time that nature allocated for the growth of an organ is over, the construction plan and the DNA instruction manual for each organ have already closed up. If our DNA did not halt these processes, humans might experience unwarranted growth spurts in any organ later in life each time the nutrient composition outside cells resembled that in the period of infant growth.

How does this relate to why infants begin storing fat? The nutrient composition of a mother's milk is relatively constant even when the mother's nutritional intake is not. However, the nutrient needs of the infant are always changing. Those nutrients most needed in the infant's body are what determine the amount of milk he or she will consume during a feeding. In other words, suckling infants effectively drink enough to acquire whatever nutrients are in lowest concentrations in the mother's milk to ensure they get enough of them. The fullness of the stomach is secondary to the infant's nutritional needs.

An infant's over-ingestion of milk will usually result in the intake of more carbohydrates than the infant needs. The carbohydrate called *lactose*, a double sugar, is the highest percentage in the composition of milk, after water. Lactose eventually breaks down to glucose, which supplies, as nature planned, the infant's energy needs throughout its body. But the excess of glucose and other elements in the milk, such as fatty acids, leads to the need for the body to store fat. In other words, fat storage occurs because we must often ingest an excess of energy nutrients while acquiring enough of the nutrients we are lacking. Since the body cannot readily excrete nutrients such as fatty acids, our body stores them in fat cells where they do not impose an immediate threat to our survival.

This theory seems to be backed up by many manifestations that the human body has adapted to survive in an environment of unpredictable nutrient supply. Consider these other adaptations our species has made that also appear to be aimed at ensuring a ready supply of nutrients:

- The stomach has the ability to accommodate different volumes of food during meals. This ability probably developed so if we needed to eat a lot of one food just to ensure we get enough of the nutrient found in the lowest amount in that food, the stomach could expand.
- The body has arranged for most fat to be stored outside the blood circulation, in our fat cells, where it otherwise would be dangerous to store (clogging arteries, etc.).
- There are no immediate untoward consequences from fat stored inside fat cells and
- Stored fat can be reconverted to fatty acids from which energy can be easily extracted.

All these adaptations suggest a highly regulated and planned system that allows humans to obtain the proper nutritional elements we need on a daily basis, even if it means that we consume an excess of one food to obtain enough nutrients during that meal.

Clarifying the Nature of Fat

It seems clear that nature never intended for the human body to consume so much food that we fill up all our fat cells, causing high levels of glucose and fatty acids to be circulating in our blood, creating the conditions for diabetes and atherosclerosis. This suggests that one of your first goals is to empty your fat cells so you can reset your body to begin burning glucose again.

Let me clarify, however, what you probably think about fat and why switching to a low-fat diet is not all that I am encouraging you to do. When we talk about fat, most people tend to think of foods that contain fats, such as meats and fish, or dairy products such as milk, butter and cheese. These are foods that break down into saturated and unsaturated fatty acids, some of which are transformed into triglycerides that end up filling your fat cells.

For decades, Americans have been led to believe that the fats we consume are the cause of heart disease and atherosclerosis. Fueled in the 1950s by research that claimed that fat clogs our arteries and leads to heart disease, the US medical community backed a campaign that blamed fats for raising low-density lipoprotein (LDL) associated cholesterol molecules that cling to cells in the lining of the blood vessels, building up to a point that they block the arteries and lead to heart attacks.

As a result of that research, doctors, nutritionists, and food gurus everywhere started promoting diets low in fat. One result was that people began substituting carbohydrates in their diets to replace the lost calories from fats. Rather than eating bacon and eggs for breakfast, many families turn to grain-based cereals (hot or cold), breads, donuts, and muffins. Smaller portions of meat for dinner are made up for with larger portions of rice, potatoes, pastas, and dinner rolls. Recipes abound that mix vegetables with pasta products and breading. In the past decade, the emphasis on "whole grain" breads, snacks, and even deserts has convinced the public that they are eating healthy. Today more than 50 percent of the average adult diet derives from carbohydrates.

There are two problems with the theory of the low-fat diet. First, some of the research about fat has been disproven and new research is furthering our knowledge that not all fat is bad. In the 1990s, researchers began to make distinctions between saturated and unsaturated fats. They noted, for example, that people in Mediterranean countries had lower, not higher, levels of heart disease, possibly due to their diets rich in fish, nuts, olives, and vegetable oils that contained up to 40% of their calories from poly- and monounsaturated fats. In the past few years, other research has shown that even saturated fats may not be as bad for the body as they have been made out to be. In addition, there are no large studies correlating saturated fats with an increased incidence of heart disease. In short, the case against dietary fat is being reevaluated, and if you hold iron-clad beliefs about fat, consider reevaluating those beliefs, too.

The second, and more important argument against a low-fat diet is that it has directly led to an explosion of diabetes. The scientific community has had a major epiphany, recognizing that carbohydrates, not fats, present the greatest danger to our health. This new scientific view completely supports my ideas that overloading your body with glucose by overeating, especially of carbohydrates, fills up your fat cells.[2] It is my observation and belief that this is precisely what causes the switch to burning fatty acids, laying the groundwork for high blood sugar and eventually diabetes.

In summary, the case against dietary fat is being reevaluated and many of the iron-clad beliefs Americans have held about avoiding foods containing fat are being reevaluated. As you follow the recommendations in this book, be aware that I do not advocate a low-fat diet if it causes you to overeat grain-based carbohydrates that give you the feeling of having a full stomach while thinking you are eating healthy.

Clarifying the HDL vs. LDL Debate

As long as we are discussing fat, let's debunk certain myths about high-density lipoproteins (HDL) and propose a new explanation for the purpose they serve. As I mentioned before, cholesterol is a fat molecule that derives from animal products. If you do not eat animal products, your liver makes cholesterol from fatty acids derived from nuts and vegetable oils.

---

[2] Time, "Ending the War on Fat," Bryan Walsh, June 23, 2014. http://time.com/2863227/ending-the-war-on-fat/

What you may not have known is that HDL and LDL proteins are also produced in the liver. The relationship between cholesterol and lipoproteins is that cholesterol molecules attach to LDL and HDL molecules, which are carried through the body. Medical science has come to call this combination of molecules 'LDL cholesterol' and 'HDL cholesterol.'

Your body needs some cholesterol, as it is used to build cell walls and make them sturdy. Without strong intestinal cell walls, your body would not be able to digest and absorb fat and you'd be running to the toilet after each meal. The relative stability of the cholesterol molecule allows the brain cells to have long-term memory. Cholesterol helps to prevent excess loss of water from the skin when the temperature outside is higher than that of the body. Cholesterol makes the skin highly resistant to chemical agents and water that might otherwise easily enter the body. The minimal solubility of cholesterol in water prevents the disintegration of the cell wall even in the presence of large amounts of water outside a cell. Cholesterol is essential to form bile salts, which promote digestion and absorption of fats in the intestine. These happen efficiently because cholesterol helps to maintain the physical integrity and malleability of cell membranes and structures inside each cell in the body.

Cholesterol molecules cannot pass through the cell walls because they have no receptor to bind onto them. However, some cholesterol molecules are attached to low-density lipoproteins, for which cell walls have specialized receptors that can bind to them. This is what allows cholesterol to pass into the cell.

When excess LDL-attached cholesterol remains in the bloodstream, it can attach to other receptors, such as in the lining of arteries, eventually building up a fatty, wax-like blockage that clogs the arteries and impedes blood flow. If this happens to arteries in the heart muscle, it can lead to a heart attack. If it happens to arteries in the brain, it can lead to a stroke. Because of this activity, LDL-cholesterol was designated as "bad" cholesterol.

Meanwhile, HDL-attached cholesterol cannot get into cells so it continuously flows through the bloodstream. The theory posits that HDL molecules are "good" because they sweep through the bloodstream collecting attached cholesterol (delivered originally as "bad" LDL-cholesterol) and returning it to the liver. In effect, the theory is that HDL molecules are cleaning agents that purify the body of attached cholesterol.

The problem is, to date, there is absolutely no proof that HDL can function this way. Moreover, it is based on implausible science. First, it is almost impossible for high-density lipoprotein to remove a cholesterol molecule that is already part of a cell because this action requires the expenditure of energy. High-density lipoprotein is only a molecule and would not have the facility to produce the energy needed to detach a cholesterol molecule from its site of attachment.

Second, even if HDL particles are able to remove the attached cholesterol, LDL can deliver another cholesterol molecule within minutes to that site because there are more LDL particles circulating in the body than HDL particles.

Given these objections, what could possibly be the value of HDL-attached cholesterol? Why would nature have evolved such that humans produce both HDL and LDL molecules to carry cholesterol through the body? The answer is highly related to other storage functions existing in the body. Just as the liver stores glucose in the form of glycogen for use in times of need for more energy, HDL-cholesterol is the liver's way of storing cholesterol for use when cells need more cholesterol. Given that cholesterol is essential to every cell in the body, HDL cholesterol in the bloodstream serves as a sort of easily accessible mobile form of storage. Since cells do not have receptors for the attachment of high-density lipoproteins, they freely float through the bloodstream, ready at any time as a reserve pool to be refitted for action, on demand. If and when cells need more cholesterol, the liver can transfer cholesterol from high-density lipoproteins into low-density lipoproteins and release them into the bloodstream for cells to use. The amount of HDL floating storage available is likely a function of each person's genetic heritage, just as it is when it comes to the amount of glucose stored as glycogen and the amount of fatty acid stored as triglyceride.

The concept of good and bad cholesterol completely misses the biological value of cholesterol, and thus misses the most important point about consuming foods containing fats. Rather than warning people to stop eating foods containing fats, the body's need for a certain amount of cholesterol suggests that ingesting cholesterol-containing foods is not the problem. The problem is *overeating these foods*, which leads to problems such as heart disease and stroke. This, of course, is not intended to question the importance of keeping LDL cholesterol level under control. That is still very important for cardiovascular health.

It's Not Fats that Make You Fat and Develop Diabetes

The case against fat is beginning to crumble, and scientists no longer view fats as the worst offender in causing disease and mortality. However, I'm not suggesting that you eat as much fatty meats and dairy as you wish. Instead, I'm proposing that you always eat what you enjoy, letting your brain guide you to the necessary nutrients. At the same time, pay conscious attention to your body's hunger and satiation signals so that you stop overeating more than your body needs to replenish itself with nutrients. The rest of this book will instruct you on how to do this.

Above all, I want you to understand that the nature of what creates fat in our body is misunderstood. The fat that fills your fat cells does not just come from the lipids in meats and dairy. Much of the fat in your fat cells derives from the glucose you consume in carbohydrates. It is the overconsumption of carbohydrates, not fats, that has led to the fastest and largest increase in prediabetes and diabetes among Americans (and people in many other countries). It is carbohydrates that we must take a new look at.

KEY POINTS

- The theory that storing fat allows us to hoard food in our bodies to protect us from periods of famine is flawed.

- The low-fat diet promoted to prevent heart disease has led many people to overconsume carbohydrates, leading to high blood sugar.

- The theory that LDL cholesterol is bad and HDL-cholesterol is good is based on implausible science. The body needs cholesterol, and LDL-cholesterol is the usable form. However, when it appears in the body in excess, it can adhere to the blood vessel wall. HDL-cholesterol is the body's way of having a readily available storehouse of cholesterol.

CHAPTER 22

Enemy #1— Our Grain-Based Culture

The last chapter discussed why nature likely set up our body to store fat, giving us the background to learn about the repercussions of the real culprit in our food chain. The biggest single filler of your fat cells are grain-based carbohydrates. These include all the complex starch foods of the grain family—wheat, oats, barley, corn, rice, rye, and others—as well as potatoes, all of which break down into glucose. (Carbs also include sucrose from fruits and lactose from milk, but we will cover those separately in the next chapter.)

The biggest threats to your health among the carbs are complex carbohydrates, particularly grains. These are the points we will cover in this chapter:

1. Carbs break down into glucose, so the more bread, pasta, rice, and potatoes you eat, the more you fill your body with glucose.
2. Most people consume far more complex carbohydrates than their body can immediately use or store.
3. Almost all of the excess glucose in your body comes from grain products, making them the most prolific cause of high blood sugar.

4. Eating "whole grain" products does nothing to mitigate the excess glucose that carbs generate in your body.

Let's now explore in detail the problems these seemingly tasty and irresistible foods cause.

The Good Side of Carbohydrates

Carbohydrates do serve a valuable purpose as the body's main source of foods that break down into glucose. Carbohydrate in the form of dissolved glucose is always present in the blood and in the fluid around cells. The normal blood glucose concentration in a person who has not eaten a meal within the past three to four hours is 90mg/dl. In a normal person, about an hour after a meal containing a large amount of carbohydrates—such as bread, pasta, rice, potatoes, or corn—the blood glucose level will seldom rise above 140 mg/dl because most of the glucose enters into the cells of the body where it is used for energy. Glucose also remains in the fluid around cells, usually in the range of 75 to 95 mg/dl, though it can fluctuate in the short term between 20 and 1500 mg/dl without any harmful consequences. If the blood glucose level falls below one-half of normal, people usually experience a loss of mental functions—confusion, forgetfulness, and lack of analytic capabilities.

Carbohydrates in the form of fructose and galactose perform specialized functions in cell membranes. For example, these sugars combine with protein or fat molecules that dangle outside cell walls and repel charged particles because of their negative charge. These combined structures attach themselves to carbohydrates protruding from other cells to maintain the cohesion of cells within an organ. These combined structures also act as receptors for binding hormones in cells and participate in our immune defense mechanisms by attacking bacteria in the blood, saliva, and tears. The identification of your blood type as A, B, AB, or O is based on the presence of these structures on the red cell wall. In addition, a special carbohydrate molecule is used in the construction of genes which reside inside the control center of each cell (the nucleus), and a variation of that molecule is used to manufacture the messenger that carries instructions from genes to workers in the cell.

Inside muscle cells, glucose that is not immediately consumed is converted to *glycogen*, an insoluble storage form of carbohydrate that can be broken down rapidly to supply energy in cells when they are low on glucose. Muscles use large amounts of glucose during exercise, especially during the early seconds of intense movement. High intensity exercise lasting 15 to 20 seconds or prolonged muscle activity (such as in endurance athletic events lasting longer than four to five hours) can completely deplete the glycogen stores in muscle. When that happens, the full restoration of glycogen in muscle usually does not occur during the next meal, as it can take up to two days or longer even if you are eating a high carbohydrate diet.

Excess glucose in the bloodstream that does not enter cells flows back into the liver, which also uses it to produce glycogen. About 120 grams of glycogen are stored in the liver for the purpose of releasing glucose back into the bloodstream to maintain a normal blood glucose level between meals.

The problem is that after the liver has made enough glycogen, whatever glucose remains is converted into triglycerides that are sent to your fat cells for storage. If your fat cells are already full, the triglycerides may accumulate in your blood. Glucose that your liver does not process also remains in your bloodstream, resulting in high blood sugar and leading to diabetes and its complications.

The complications of diabetes occur because a significant and lasting rise in blood glucose, like that occurring in diabetes, can lead to the attachment of glucose molecules to different proteins in the body. This process is called *glycation*. The body can tolerate a certain amount of glycation without experiencing ill effects. However, too much glycation can lead to the impairment of cell function in organs such as kidneys and the brain. It is thought that Alzheimer's disease starts with glycation of proteins in the brain, peripheral neuropathy (deadening of the nerves) with glycation of proteins around the nerves in the leg, and cataracts with glycation of proteins in the lens of the eye.

How Much Carbohydrate Do We Need?

The body needs some carbohydrates, but the question is, how much? It depends to some extent on your age and level of activity.

During infancy and childhood, our carbohydrate needs are very high relative to our body size because we are rapidly growing cells in almost every organ. A developing infant's body requires an abundance of energy to duplicate cell walls and internal structures. Our cells are on an unending process to replicate themselves, taking their instructions from growth hormone released from the pituitary gland. Cell division is like splitting a house into two, with each half being transformed into a new house with its own walls, appliances, plumbing, wiring, waste disposal and heating. Those houses then split in two yet again, as the cell division process continues.

As you approach adulthood, you need less glucose for two reasons. First, your cells multiply more slowly because new cells are mostly formed to replace dead cells within organs, rather than to build new structures. As a result, there is reduced glucose need for cell division. As you age, there is usually a reduction in muscle mass, so there are fewer cells where glucose can be stored as muscle glycogen. Reduced muscle mass also means reduced energy needs.

As a general rule, you can think of the answer to this question in this way: *the quantity of carbohydrate consumed during a meal should not be more than what you need to replenish the glycogen stores in your liver and muscles, unless you are exercising immediately after a meal. Any excess carbohydrate that remains in the body is what your liver converts into triglycerides that are stored in your fat cells. When your fat cells are full, the excess glucose remains in your bloodstream.*

This means that if you tend to be sedentary, you don't need many complex carbohydrates. No one can give you a specific recommendation on quantity, but if you get in touch with your authentic weight, you will sense how reducing your carbohydrate intake helps you lose weight and maintain your weight loss.

Carbohydrates Fool Your Taste Buds

Since the body needs only a certain amount of carbohydrates, it is perhaps not ironic that most complex carbs come from bland foods. Perhaps nature is telling us not to eat too much carbohydrate. If you have ever eaten bread, rice, corn, or potatoes without any salt, butter, or seasonings, you know how lacking in taste they are.

The reason complex carbohydrates taste bland is that when you chew them, they break down into molecules that are too large to fit into the taste receptors in the mouth. In order to fit, a complex carbohydrate molecule has to be broken down to the size of a double sugar unit. ("Complex" carbohydrates are called complex because they are composed of more than two sugar molecule units.) An enzyme present in saliva begins that breakdown process, but in general, complex carbohydrate molecules stay in the mouth only long enough to convert less than 5 percent of all their molecules into double sugar units. If you alter your chewing speed, you can increase the release of double sugar units. Further breakdown of complex carbs into double sugar units happens in the intestine, where an exocrine enzyme from the pancreas knocks the molecules apart.

What you taste when you eat food containing complex carbohydrates are actually the vitamins and minerals your nutrient-counting brain has come to associate with that particular carbohydrate, as well as any spices, sugar, salt, oil or fat added to it. This means that in reality, you are enjoying only a tiny portion of the complex carbohydrates you eat. You're unlikely to be aware of this because you typically eat foods with complex carbohydrates topped with gravy, sauce, butter, syrup, jam, jelly, salt, seasonings, or other condiments. Without these, you would taste almost nothing from bread, rice, potatoes, pasta, and other grain-based foods.

Serious Disadvantages of Consuming Complex Carbs

You may not be aware of this when you eat (or overeat) complex carbs, but you are actually doing your body a disservice. Given that the receptors on your taste buds cannot register the large molecules in complex carbs, and the molecules are not volatile and so are not carried by air to your smell receptors, the normal digestive processes do not fully kick in. When you chew other foods, the nutrient molecules fit into the receptors of your taste buds, like the teeth of one gear wheel fitting into the slot of another. This triggers the release of signals telling the brain what nutrients are present. The brain then begins releasing the right mix of enzymes into your saliva and in the intestines to help digest these nutrients properly.

If you are eating a meal with a lot of complex carbohydrate content, however, the sheer number of large molecules interferes with and even overpowers the presence of the other nutrient molecules on your taste bud receptors. This not only dampens your appreciation of the flavors of the other foods and their nutrients, but interferes with your brain's command of the digestive processes. Your inability to enjoy bites of complex carbohydrates and their interference with the enjoyment of other nutrients prompts you to swallow quickly in anticipation of enjoying the next bite of food. Through repetition of this process over years, you end up eating your meals faster and faster while enjoying less of what you eat. This also tends to fool you into consuming more food if it is in front of you. Over time, without realizing what is happening, you become a fast eater who craves a lot of carbohydrates.

Is this characterization true for you? When you eat bread, do you pay attention to the bread itself or to the butter, mayo, mustard, or other condiment slathered on it? When you eat a sandwich or a sub for lunch, do you tend to take a bite, chew it fast and eagerly swallow so you can "taste" the next bite? When you eat rice, corn, or potatoes, especially mashed potatoes, don't you tend to gobble them down and swallow fast with hardly any chewing? Do you often get stomachaches, a bloated feeling, or indigestion when you eat meals with lots of carbs? This is because your digestive juices are not properly mixed to handle the amount of carbs you have consumed.

Many people develop the "speedy eating" habit and rationalize it away by saying they eat fast because of time constraints, or argue that they were going to consume the entire meal anyway, so what difference does it make how fast they eat it?

The World's Plentiful Grains: The Scourge of Diabetes

The ancestors of modern humans appeared on earth about 50,000 years ago. Cultivation of plants started only after 40,000 years of human existence. The domestication of rice and grains like wheat and rye dates back to only about 13,000 to 10,000 BCE. This means that humans survived without consuming significant amounts of grain and grain products for a majority of human history.

Humans were always equipped to break down complex carbohydrates, as the presence of *amylase* in the intestine, the enzyme that digests complex carbohydrates, shows. But it's likely that early humans obtained complex carbohydrates and carbohydrate associated nutrients from vegetables that required chewing such as yam, cassava, potato, and taro. The consumption of grain and grain-based food products is not necessary for human well-being.

It was not until several millennia ago that carbohydrate from grains became a staple of the human diet. In the middle ages, many cultures survived on porridge, rice, or potatoes depending on which crops grew in their region. In the late 19th century, industrialized roller mills were invented, making it easier to refine grains into flour and other products made with starches and flours. Because of this, grains became the major source of carbohydrate in human diets.

Today, modern agricultural practices allow us to cultivate hybridized, drought-resistant crops using irrigation, fertilizer and machinery to produce an abundance of carbohydrates to feed humanity. The top three crops produced in the world are rice, maize and wheat. Each is cultivated at a level of 600 to 800 million tons per year in order to feed billions of people around the globe and to provide nutrition for the animals we eat.

In general, grains are easy to transport, fast to cook, easy to chew and easily digested and absorbed (except by people with celiac disease or grain allergies). Milling grains to create flour makes them easy to store without refrigeration. Refining produces starches and flours with qualities that chefs can exploit to create a multitude of dishes and products. For example, wheat can be refined into flour with a high protein content to make crusty or chewy breads, or a low protein content suitable for cakes, cookies, and piecrusts. Wheat flour is also used to thicken gravy and sauces. The variety of edible products that can be made with the carbohydrate from grains is never ending, and we are tempted by these food items throughout the world.

This triumvirate of corn, wheat and rice has become the primary source of energy for humans worldwide. They provide glucose energy for our brains and muscles and facilitate the production of triglycerides that we store as fat for later use as our fuel.

It is thus not surprising to see the increasing incidence of weight gain and associated conditions such as Type 2 diabetes in regions of the world where easily digestible grain-based carbohydrates are the main staple. According to a 2014 analysis of health survey data, individuals born between the years 1966 to 1980 are twice as likely to have diabetes compared to individuals of the same age born between 1946 and 1965.[1]

In the US, one of the major factors behind our love for carbohydrates arose out of the misguided war against fat. As discussed in the last chapter, in the mid-1980s, a million Americans were dying from heart disease, believed to be caused by the consumption of fatty foods. Politicians declared war on this public health issue. Scientists identified low density lipoprotein (LDL) cholesterol as the villain. The National Institutes of Health recommended that all Americans eat less fat and cholesterol to reduce the risk of heart disease.

In response, the food industry promulgated the virtues of "healthy" carbohydrates over fats. Americans bought into this science and increased their intake of carbohydrate while reducing their consumption of fat. Grain-based cereals for breakfast, sandwiches for lunch and rice, potatoes or corn to accompany dinners became staples of the American diet, along with mass-produced donuts, cakes, pies and breads. The result: the prevalence of Type 2 diabetes increased over 160 percent from 1980 to 2012.

As mentioned, carbohydrate intake now accounts for over 50 percent of the calories in the typical adult diet in the US. Even the USDA recommends multiple servings of grains per day. Many expert panels encourage the consumption of "whole" grain products, believing in their health benefits just because they contain B vitamins, vitamin E and fiber normally associated with bran. The medical community further aids this process with pronouncements exalting the virtues of eating the first meal—usually some grain-based cereal, oatmeal, or bread—that gets you ready for the day. They emphasize this directive by warning that those who don't have breakfast are likely to consume a mid-morning snack containing more energy than they would have consumed at breakfast.

The food industry has been happy to exploit this opportunity by marketing easy-to-prepare cereals and many grain-based products for breakfast. The food companies even procure endorsements from medical associations and experts

---

[1] *Are Baby Boomers Healthier than Generation X? A Profile of Australia's Working Generations Using National Health Survey Data.* Pilkington et al. PLoS One 9(3): March 2014

regarding products made with whole grains, the virtues of the vitamins, minerals, and proteins they have added to grain-based products, or the deletion of particles such as gluten from these products. Focusing on these supposed health benefits in their advertising has made it easier for the general population to completely overlook the serious impact that the carbs in these food have on their blood glucose levels.

This cavalier attitude towards the medically unsound nature of excessive carbohydrate diets has given food manufacturers ammunition to entice the general population to consume more and more grain-based foods: bagels, baguettes, breadsticks, buns, croissants, pretzels and rolls; challah, chapatti, focaccia, injera, lavash, naan, paratha, pita, pizza and tortilla; bhatura, frybread, puri and sopaipilla; biscuits, cakes, crackers, cupcakes, doughnuts, muffins and pastries; mantou, pot stickers, dumplings, noodles and other pastas; crepes, pan, pancakes, pandesal, pies, and other food products prepared with grain flours using ethnic cuisines and regional flavors.

These all sound so good, don't they? But eating them may be putting you at risk of high blood sugar and diabetes.

Chemical Composition of Carbohydrates

To truly understand the health impact of grain-based complex carbohydrates, it helps to know what carbohydrate molecules are. Complex carbohydrate is made by creating a bond between carbon atom number 1 of one glucose molecule and carbon atom number 4 of another glucose molecule (figure 16).

COMPLEX CARBOHYDRATE

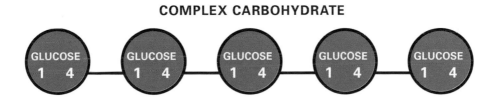

Figure 16. Complex carbohydrate is made by creating a bond between carbon atom number 1 of one glucose molecule and carbon atom number 4 of another glucose molecule. They are too large to be sensed by sugar receptors on the taste cells.

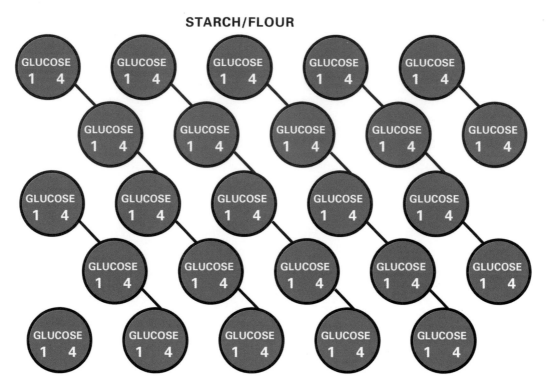

STARCH/FLOUR

Figure 17. Starch is made out of glucose molecules linked to each other in complex ways. Each molecule of flour (starch) may contain up to 200,000 glucose molecules, branching every 24 to 30 units and tightly packed. Consumption of starch from grains is responsible for the sustained elevation of your blood sugar (glucose) level.

Similarly, starch (a form of complex carbohydrate) is composed of long strings of glucose with branches that also have long strings of glucose (figure 17). Thousands of glucose molecules can bond together in these long strings. The process is something like the way polycarbonate solid plastic is made by combining carbonate units together. When you bond carbonate units to each other, they get stronger and can be molded into many shapes such as tubes, rods, and sheets, each with different properties of rigidity and heat tolerance.

You can alter the properties of the starch by varying how the glucose molecules branch off from the main chain. Wheat, corn, and rice products are effectively large chains of glucose molecules that are neatly folded and tightly compressed to form starches of different solubility, clarity, and responsiveness to chemical and physical conditions. These starches and flours can be used to make numerous dishes.

Your body has to break down starch to simpler chains of molecules to end up with glucose molecules that can enter your cells. As mentioned, your liver also converts glucose into glycogen, which is the body's storage form of starch. Glycogen is a much simpler chain of molecules, with branches every 8 to 12 glucose units compared to every 24 to 30 glucose units in naturally occurring starch. This simpler structure allows glycogen to be broken down rapidly in both liver cells and muscles by enzymes activated by adrenaline when the body needs a surge of energy.

All carbohydrates are effectively sugar. It doesn't matter whether they are whole grain or refined in any way. When you pick up two pieces of bread, buns, or rolls to make a sandwich, you are holding long chains of sugar molecules baked to stay firm so you can grasp them. When you flatten dough to make pizza or flat bread, you are shaping sugar into sheets. When you cook noodles and pasta, you are cooking sugar shaped into strings, strips, tubes, shells or wings. When you make a waffle on a waffle iron or a pancake on a frying pan, you are pouring sugar batter to make specific formations. The cookie you hold is a piece of sugar sculpture. The mound of rice on your bowl or plate is a heap of sugar.

You would probably never consume a bowl of sugar, soaked with milk, with or without added fruits and/or nuts. Yet this is what you are basically eating when the bowl contains breakfast cereal made from whole grain, and manufactured to camouflage the sugar molecules. When you eat complex carbohydrate products like a sandwich or pasta, you seldom think that you are eating sugar. When you dip vegetables, fish, shrimp or meat in a batter of grain flour you are coating them with sugar. But this is effectively what you are doing—eating food that becomes glucose in your blood.

Remember this: each 4 grams of carbohydrates you eat is about 1 teaspoon of sugar.

Check the comparisons below to see the equivalent amount of sugar you are eating in your ordinary foods.

Product	Serving size	Carbohydrate (grams)	Actual Sugar Content (teaspoons)
Bread	1 slice	12	3
Breakfast cereal	1 cup	30	7½
12" sandwich roll (like a sub or hoagie)	1 roll	36	9
Pizza	1 slice	40	10
Pasta	2 ounces	40	10
Rice	1 cup	48	12
Bagel	1	48	12

Reasons We Lose Control of Our Carb Intake

Given the preponderance of carbs in our lives, most adults consume more than they need for immediate energy production and glycogen restoration in the liver. There are many reasons for overconsumption. If you're serious about getting back to your authentic weight, decide which of the following reasons apply to you and act accordingly to reduce your carbohydrate intake.

Childhood patterns and associations. Many adults eat carbohydrates according to patterns of intake formed in their childhood. For example, you may eat a lot of crackers and snack foods between meals, or bread and dinner rolls with your meals, or you may accompany every main course with rice or potatoes, just as your family did. Perhaps you put croutons in your salads as your Mom did, or use flatbread to pick up the meat or vegetables, as many Asian, African, and Middle Eastern cultures do. These patterns can be so ingrained that they seem natural and you feel you can't live without them. You do them without thinking and do not correlate these patterns with excess glucose consumption. The way you eat was part of your upbringing and supported by parents, families, and the social customs of your culture.

Eating too fast for your brain to assess your nutritional intake. Carbohydrate that is soft, blended, or pureed and doesn't require much chewing, such as soft bread or cooked rice, moves quickly through the mouth, as if being suctioned into the stomach by a vacuum cleaner. If the carbohydrate you eat requires minimal or no chewing, you are likely to swallow it faster and eat the meal more quickly compared to another food that requires more chewing. The faster a food moves through the mouth, the less contact it has with the taste buds. Also, as mentioned, starch molecules do not fit into the receptors of sweet-sensing taste buds so the brain lacks information about what nutrients are incoming. This means that your brain's regulatory system is unable to determine when to tell you to stop intake based on your internal nutritional need. If you are in the habit of consuming all of the food on your plate, including all the carbohydrates, your quantity control is very likely quite arbitrary. You will eat whatever is placed in front of you, with no distinction between too much carbohydrate and just enough.

Lack of accurate information from food producers. Many of the micronutrients associated with natural fiber, a complex carbohydrate, have still not been identified, and the Recommended Daily Amount (RDA) has not yet been ascertained. Even when scientists identify the micronutrients and quantify the RDA for them, the RDA depends on each person's individual chemistry. It is unlikely that commercial preparations of foods will contain the amount of RDA that each person needs. Only your brain knows what specific vitamins, minerals, and nutrients your body is deficient in at any given time. Based on past experience, your brain also knows which foods can supply those. Thus, if you don't regularly consume enough natural fiber from fruits and vegetables, your brain often directs you through intuition and craving to consume grain-based carbohydrate to acquire the needed amounts of micronutrients.

Many food manufacturers use carbohydrate-based fat replacers to produce a familiar texture, appearance, and taste in food while reducing the fat content of their products so they can promote them as low-fat, healthy alternatives. Some of these replacers, such as modified starches and dextrins, are digested in the intestine, adding to the amount of carbohydrate available for absorption.

Compensating for a deficit in nutritional value. You may be eating too much carbohydrate because your brain believes it can extract more nutrient value from these foods, but the nutrients are lacking. For example, to produce energy from glucose, cells need not only oxygen, but micronutrients such as B vitamins. In nature, B vitamins are present in whole grains and foods such as potatoes, bananas, lentils, chili peppers, and beans. However, today's cultivation and refining process of whole grains often depletes them of a significant portion of micronutrients like B vitamins. This could make you crave more carbohydrate, because your brain believes it can derive more Vitamin B from it. Taking a vitamin or mineral supplement might actually help you reduce this craving, though you have to be careful to choose a supplement that does not contain levels above the Recommended Daily Allowance of some vitamins or minerals.

Your brain is craving a specific nutrient. If your brain has identified a particular carbohydrate-based food preparation as the source of a vitamin or mineral because that is how the body received them while you were growing up, you could experience craving to consume that particular food preparation in order to get the needed nutrient. For example, if grits was the source for niacin in your childhood, you'll crave grits if your body is deficient in that vitamin when you're an adult. Similarly, if you habitually obtained certain nutrients through fruit juices instead of natural fruits, you might experience a craving for fruit juices.

False sensation of 'feeling' full. Overconsumption feeds on itself. In other words, once you start overeating for any of the above reasons, your stomach becomes used to the feeling of being full after eating. Carbs especially provide that sensation of being full because the mash made from carbs in your mouth expands many times in your stomach when mixed with liquid. Relying on the fullness of the stomach as the signal to stop eating often initiates carbohydrate over-consumption as a means to feel full. This reinforces the feeling that your meal is not over until you feel that same sense of fullness.

Alternating high and low blood sugar syndrome. Your mouth begins detecting sugar molecules immediately upon eating, which triggers the release of insulin in your body during a meal to deal with the flood of glucose that will soon be in your bloodstream. Normally the glucose is absorbed in your cells within two to four hours after a meal. But a meal high in carbohydrate content can lead to higher insulin levels. If the insulin release is robust in response to the surge in your blood sugar, the glucose will be quickly removed from the blood, rapidly lowering the blood sugar level to an amount that creates feelings of fatigue. This is one reason why many people feel tired a few hours after breakfast and lunch, leading them to snack on foods containing more carbohydrate because they feel they need more sugar. This syndrome can create a vicious cycle and cause weight gain.

Feeling pressure over time or not paying attention. Many people overeat carbohydrates simply because they let other conditions influence their pace of eating. For example, when dining with friends and family, you typically pay close attention to the conversation and don't realize how much food you're consuming until you have eaten too much. There are also occasions when you have only a limited time to finish a meal you paid for, are afraid that you won't get a chance to eat again soon enough, or don't want to waste food or offend a gracious host who has cooked up a huge batch of pasta, rice, or potatoes. As a result, you consume more carbohydrate-based food.

Sweet tooth syndrome. Many people develop a craving for something sweet after a meal, but desserts like cakes and pies are prepared with grain flour and sugar. This carbohydrate adds to those you may have eaten during the meal itself. Eating more carbohydrate in the name of having something sweet can only lead to the absorption of more sugar.

Craving for salt. If carbohydrate-based foods are the main source for salt in your body, you might crave and consume more carbohydrate if your body is used to having a high salt content. In the next chapter we will examine how salt content in the foods you eat influences the intake of carbohydrate.

Recommendations to Control Your Carb Intake

In theory, it should be easy to reduce your intake of grains and grain products compared to the amount you consume now. It is generally easy to identify and isolate grain and grain products during a meal and not eat them. However, in practice, cutting back can be very difficult because it requires you to change routines that you have probably had since childhood. In addition, you see the same pattern of eating grains and grain products among many people around you—your parents, grandparents, family members, friends, acquaintances, and even strangers. Grains are a staple of the diet in nearly every culture and so are difficult to avoid.

Therefore, you need a clear and compelling reason to significantly alter your eating habits to reduce your intake of complex carbohydrates. Because grains and grain products are the most likely sources for the majority of carbohydrate in your diet, substantially reducing their intake is the best way to reduce your intake of carbohydrate. There is no way around it but to admit that your own voluntary choice to reduce carbohydrate intake is essential to maintaining your authentic weight, health, and well-being.

To help myself reduce carbohydrate intake, I think of grains as food intended for birds and animals. Visualizing it this way may help you shun grains, seeing yourself as a bird pecking away at a bowl of rice or pasta. In addition, remember that since cooked grains and grain products are not very tasty by themselves, notice how much you're obliged to consume salt, refined sugar, butter or other ingredients to give them some taste appeal.

Below are five ways you can immediately begin lowering your consumption of carbohydrates.

1. Suck on a hard mint when you feel hungry. You will find your craving to eat will almost always subside if you pop a mint in your mouth and slowly suck on it. We know this works because it solves the problem for diabetics who develop hypoglycemia (low blood sugar). As soon as they ingest about 15 grams of sugar (in their case, they often take glucose tablets), they experience rapid relief of symptoms such as altered mental functions, palpitation, sweating, and hunger.

How can a little mint or glucose tablet help, given that it is such a small amount of sugar, insufficient to alter their blood sugar level? It seems more likely that the quickness of relief suggests a mechanism not based on absorbing sugar but rather on the fact that the taste buds, in registering molecules of sugar, reassure the brain that glucose is on the way. The brain then moderates the symptoms that were intended to alert the individual of the need for sugar and the developing symptoms of hypoglycemia recede. You can do the same by stimulating your tongue with a mint candy. In research tests, just 100 milligrams of sugar resulted in reducing the intensity of hunger in subjects.

2. Stop eating grains and carbs that don't need to be chewed. Avoid eating complex carbohydrates that do not need to be chewed very much or that you tend to quickly eat and swallow. Eliminate rice, mashed potatoes, breads made with grains, corn-based products, and foods that have been blended with any starches from your diet. Replace them with edible tubers and roots such as whole potatoes, tapioca, taro and yams prepared in a way that allows you to chew them. These types of foods will provide your body with fiber and fiber-associated nutrients in their natural form.

For a person with elevated blood sugar, the best source of carbohydrate is lentils. Fibers naturally present in lentils take longer to digest and thus result in a much slower elevation of blood sugar after your meal, compared to consuming grain products that digest quickly. This means less insulin release, slower removal of sugar from the blood, no feelings of nervousness, trembling, or tiredness and thus no need to snack a few hours after breakfast or lunch.

3. Chew all your food more slowly. As you chew, you are warming and mixing the nutrients, releasing their molecules so they can attach to the taste buds and be carried to the smell receptors in the nose, resulting in signals to the brain. The brain, in turn, translates these signals into a pleasing eating experience, similar to how your ears create a pleasing listening experience by combining signals generated by your ear drums when you hear notes of music played by different sections of an orchestra. Slow chewing helps your brain regulate your digestive process and provides you with the signal to stop eating when you've had enough nutrient intake. In one study, hungry participants ate an average of 13 grams less carbohydrate when they paid attention to taste sensations during a meal compared to their normal intake.

4. Little by little, leave an increasing amount of food on your plate. This is a simple little experiment of your will power. Start by leaving 1/8 of the food, then 2/8, and finally up to 1/3 of the food served to you. This test will allow you to investigate what signals it takes to give your digestive system the sense of satisfaction. Of course, the most useful foods to leave on the plate are the carbohydrates made from grains. If rice, pasta, bread, or mashed potatoes have been served, push them aside. By eating fewer grain and grain-based foods, you will enjoy your meals more and will be surprised to find that soon after the meal, you'll feel completely satisfied without having experienced the sense of fullness you used to have at the end of a meal that included grains. You'll also realize that you still have the same level of energy you had when eating a lot of carbohydrates from grains.

5. Add herbs and spices to all your dishes. When you eat an energy-containing food such as grits to obtain niacin, as mentioned earlier, your body has to deal with the other nutrients in grits. This means the body will be seeking more micronutrients to metabolize the extra carbohydrate the body was forced to absorb. Your brain, in turn, may look to a familiar source for the solution and thus you eat even more carbohydrate than before.

One way to get around this vicious cycle is by finding an alternate source for micronutrients. One of the best sources for these are natural spices and herbs that come from different parts of plants. The use of spices and herbs in cooking started in at least 2000 BCE. It is thought that our ancestors used spices after discovering that they helped prevent spoilage of food. While our ancestors did not understand why, it is the antimicrobial properties that make spices a useful food ingredient, especially in warmer climates, where infectious diseases can be spread through meat, which is particularly susceptible to spoiling. However, this doesn't explain the extensive use of spices in a country like India, where much of the population is vegetarian, and their use in Mediterranean cultures that use a lot of fresh seafood.

My explanation for mankind's use of spices in cooking comes back to the brain's regulatory mechanism. I suggest that spices are used to make meals more enjoyable because, in the brain, this enjoyment signifies the arrival of a needed micronutrient in the mouth. The evidence for this lies in the fact that spices and herbs contain abundant vitamins, minerals, and antioxidants in significant portions that make them ideal sources of micronutrients. In fact, herbs and spices can be the source of at least 25 percent of the nutrients listed in Chapter 11.

One of the observations I have made after studying how people eat and its relationship to diabetes is that people who live in cultures that use a lot of spices in their cooking tend to eat less. This is because the enjoyment of spices comes from the nutrients contained in them. People who eat spiced foods do not have to consume a lot of energy nutrients just to get the essential nutrients they need. If you eat a meal cooked with spices, you will not only enjoy the taste, but may eat less rice, potatoes, bread, and even less meat because the spices provide you with needed micronutrients.

If this is true, then why is the incidence of Type 2 diabetes increasing at an alarming rate in places like India and China? Just as in the US, there is a significant increase in the consumption of grains and grain-based foods heavily marketed by food and agribusinesses. In the name of profits, corporate food companies now market mass-produced food items made with large amounts of starches and salt in these countries. Fast food restaurants have also become ubiquitous, especially in large urban areas.

If you are developing prediabetes and are accustomed to eating spices, all you need to do is return to eating your meals seasoned with more spices, while gradually subtracting grain and grain products from your diet. This will prevent your progression to diabetes. If you are not used to a variety of spices, gradually incorporate herbs and spices into your diet while weaning yourself of grain and grain products.

KEY POINTS

- The problem with glucose is that any excess that cells cannot burn or that the liver cannot convert to glycogen (stored in the liver) or to triglycerides (stored in fat cells) ends up in the bloodstream. This leads to the attachment of glucose molecules to different proteins in the body (called glycation), initiating the damaging complications of diabetes.

- Whole grains are composed of starch made out of glucose molecules linked to each other in complex ways, but they are effectively sugar.

- Identify the reasons you eat or overeat grains and grain-based products. Then apply the many techniques proposed to reduce your intake.

Since implementing the recommendations of EAT CHEW LIVE to eliminate grain-based carbohydrates and eat mindfully, I have lost 14 pounds and my A1C has declined significantly. When I went off my new regimen, my weight went up and my A1C climbed back up. I now understand the importance of sticking to the recommendations. I feel so much healthier as I approach my authentic weight.

Rick, Prediabetic, California

CHAPTER 23

Natural Sugar vs. Glucose

Many people are confused about whether natural sugar, i.e., sucrose, is the same as glucose in your bloodstream. This form of sugar is found in fruit, berries, sugar cane, sugar beets, and other crops that can be boiled down into forms of sugar. The confusion is understandable because, when discussing diabetes, we always refer to the problem of having high blood 'sugar.' The same word 'sugar' appears to be referring to the same item, so there is a tendency to think that eating any natural sugar increases your blood sugar. For example, many people make pastries with reduced amounts of sugar (sucrose) believing that they can now consume more of them, without realizing that they may be actually consuming more sugar (glucose) from the flour used.

But digesting natural sugar is not the same as filling your bloodstream with glucose. Sucrose contains equal parts of glucose and fructose (figure 18). Both are absorbed as they're released in the intestine. But while the glucose adds to your blood sugar level almost immediately, fructose is absorbed only half as fast as glucose and has to be further processed into glucose before it can elevate your blood sugar level. This means eating a piece of fruit doesn't add the same amount of glucose to your bloodstream as quickly as eating an equal amount of carbohydrate in mashed potatoes or bread.

The same is true for milk sugar (*lactose*), which is made of 1 molecule of galactose and 1 molecule of glucose. Galactose must be further processed by the liver before it can elevate your blood sugar. The medical profession has done a poor job of educating people that natural sugar has not been shown to increase the incidence of complications in Type 2 diabetes. In fact, the medical profession may have unwittingly contributed to creating a prevailing culture in which people fear the natural sugars of whole fruit.

NATURAL SUGARS

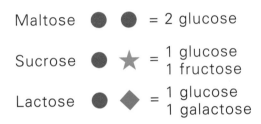

Figure 18. Natural sugars are either two linked-up single sugar molecules, as shown, or single sugar molecules such as fructose.

The human experience with natural sugar started when our hunter-gatherer ancestors experienced the sweetness of berries and fruits, possibly because the sweet taste indicated that the food was safe. Our experience with sweet taste starts as a baby when we consume lactose, the milk sugar, or regular sugar. When any of these sugars come into contact with the sweet-sensing taste buds in the mouth, it sends signals to the brain which produces the sensation of sweetness.

Because there is some glucose in natural sugars, the brain causes the release of insulin from the pancreas. This facilitates the transfer of glucose already in the blood into cells in the body to make room for the glucose expected to be absorbed from the gut. Elevation of blood sugar after the digestion and absorption of food reassures the brain that glucose has been received as expected, a state of starvation has been averted, and fuel in the form of glucose is available for immediate or future use. Through repetition of this experience, when any type of sugar stimulates the sweet-sensing taste buds, it produces a pleasing response because your brain has a learned experience of satisfaction based on nutritive value. Over time, the body associates the sweet taste with the imminent arrival of glucose in the blood. This is similar to you receiving a paycheck. From experience, you know what it represents—soon to be available money in your bank account.

In short, eating a piece of fruit for breakfast or as a dessert does not deliver the same immediate glucose impact to your blood as eating a grain-based product such as toast, muffins, cake, or pie, so it is effectively healthier for you.

To Use No-calorie Sweeteners or Not?

Many people believe that consuming no-calorie sweeteners reduces their intake of energy from natural sugars in food. However, there are many reasons why this is a misleading and counterproductive idea.

First, certain molecules of no-calorie sweeteners act through a separate receptor on the sweet-sensing taste buds on your tongue to send signals to the brain. These molecules do not contain any energy the body can use, but the brain interprets the signals as if they do and generates the sensation of sweetness. Based on previous experiences with the sweet sensation from natural sugars such as lactose, sucrose, and maltose, the brain expects that there will soon be glucose to be absorbed. When none enters the body, however, the brain can become confused and ultimately change its interpretation of the sensation of sweetness. This is like depositing your paycheck only to find out that the check does not represent money because the issuer's bank account did not have sufficient funds. After that experience, you begin attaching no importance to any future check you get from that issuer.

The brain's inability to accurately predict what should happen to your blood glucose levels after the sweet taste buds have been stimulated could eventually cause it to misinterpret the consumption of real carbohydrate during a meal. This misinterpretation can delay the generation of the satisfaction signal that occurs when the intensity of enjoyment is reduced—an important factor in regulating your food intake during a meal (as you will learn in Chapter 30). In addition, it could also delay the release of insulin and other hormones to manage the high levels of blood sugar that occur when you eat a meal loaded with complex carbohydrates.

Second, based on the false assumption that you're being "good" when you use sweetness from a no-calorie sweetener to eat more of a carbohydrate preparation, you're actually being 'penny wise and pound foolish' because your blood sugar can go higher than it would have otherwise.

Third, the prolonged use of a no-calorie sweetener could cause you to lose the sensation of sweetness when you eat naturally sweet edibles such as fruits. To compensate, you might eventually begin adding no-calorie sweeteners to these, creating a 'not sweet enough' syndrome. If you put two teaspoons of sugar in your mouth, the sweetness you experience is not double that of one teaspoon of sugar. This effect is similar to how your other senses behave. For example, ten people singing the same note will not be perceived as being ten times louder than one person singing the note. In other words, loudness does not increase proportionately with the number of people singing. In the same way, once you become accustomed to the intensity of sweetness of a no-calorie sweetener, the taste of natural sugar in fruits may not be perceived as providing adequate sweetness because of the way your mechanism of taste perception works.

A fourth problem with no-calorie sweeteners is that they are often substituted for sugar in recipes for sweets such as desserts. This leads people to believe it is okay to eat these foods since they contain no sugar. However, most desserts are also loaded with calories from butter, cream, nuts, and other ingredients. In this case, the purpose of eating sweets with no-calorie sweeteners and no added sugar to reduce energy intake is defeated by the presence of other energy nutrients.

Yet another problem is that the use of no-calorie sweetener can indirectly spur a craving to consume complex carbohydrates when your brain senses a significant lowering of blood sugar. In the past, the brain believed that it could expect glucose absorption soon after experiencing the sweet sensation. But the meaning of the sweet taste has been usurped. Your brain therefore may prompt you to eat a complex carbohydrate to make up for the missing glucose because the mouth feel of complex carbohydrate and subsequent expectation of arrival of glucose in the blood remain intact. This can turn into a cycle of consuming no-calorie sweetened foods followed by a craving for real carbohydrates and increased risk of Type 2 diabetes.[1]

The Plague of High Sugar Content Drinks

There is a literal pandemic of beverages and foods now produced with added sugar or high-fructose corn syrup. These are well-known taste-enhancing additives that increase the palatability, presentation, aroma, and texture of food to make consumers want to eat more than they need in a serving. The proof of this is in the astonishing statistic that Americans consume an average of 22 teaspoons of added sugar per day, most of it in the form of soda and sweetened drinks. You may not realize the enormous amount of sugar in many of these drinks. While an eight ounce glass of milk contains about three teaspoons of natural sugar, there are eight teaspoons of sugar in a can of regular soda.

These beverages are often consumed in response to thirst when the brain expects receptors in the mouth to experience water molecules. If the sugar concentration in such beverages were similar to that of a natural beverage, such as milk, the body would be able to regulate the sugar consumed. But if the beverage you consume is sweetened with sugar or an energy-containing sweetener at a concentration above what is natural, the brain has no mechanism to regulate how much you need to drink to satisfy your thirst based on the experience of sweet taste. You are then forced to terminate drinking based either on a feeling of fullness in your stomach or the emptiness of the container. This is why many people tend to drink large amounts of soft drinks or sweetened juices when they are thirsty, adding to their increased consumption of sugar.

I recommend weaning yourself off sodas and beverages with added sugar or high-fructose corn syrup to reduce your intake of carbohydrates.

---

[1] Swithers SE 2013, Artificial sweeteners produce the counterintuitive effect of inducing metabolic derangements. Trends in Endocrinology and Metabolism. 24:431-441

Beers, Wines and Spirits
(distilled beverages)

Typically, beers, wines and spirits contain between 3 and 40 percent of ethanol (alcohol) by volume. The molecules of alcohol you consume are changed in the liver. The resulting chemicals can be inserted into the same metabolic line that uses glucose for energy production. This means that glucose molecules that would normally have been used for energy production remain unused, leaving them in the liver or bloodstream. In addition, beers and wines also contain sugars that contribute glucose. This explains why the body may convert almost all the excess glucose to fat to be stored in available areas—think beer belly—as well as contributing to high blood sugar.

When people drink alcohol, especially in a social setting, they also tend to munch on something that contains carbohydrates. This means that consuming alcohol can be a double whammy to your carb consumption if you are prediabetic or diabetic.

KEY POINTS

- Natural sugar (sucrose) contains equal parts of glucose and fructose, which the liver must break down into glucose. This means eating a piece of fruit doesn't add the same amount of glucose to your bloodstream as fast as eating mashed potatoes or bread.

- When any type of sugar stimulates the sweet-sensing taste buds, it produces a pleasing response because your brain has a learned experience of satisfaction based on the nutritive value of glucose arriving in the blood.

- Consuming no-calorie sweeteners can confuse the brain into believing glucose will be arriving and end up throwing off your natural mechanisms of regulation of carbohydrate intake.

CHAPTER 24

The Role of Salt in Diabetes

In any conversation about diabetes, the only issue that seems to come up is sugar. However, high salt intake is one of the contributing factors to high blood sugar and diabetes. The way in which salt interacts with your cells is complex, but I hope you will take the time to read this chapter, because reducing your salt intake is crucial to lowering your blood sugar level.

The Story of Salt

For most of human history, the typical diet was low in sodium because sodium was not plentiful. In ancient Rome, most salt was dug out of salt mines by prisoners and slaves because the mining work was dangerous. Constant contact with rock salt and breathing salt dust shortened the lives of the miners. Salt was so valuable that Roman soldiers were either paid with salt or a 'salarium' to buy salt; hence our English word 'salary.'

Some civilizations also learned to evaporate salt from the ocean in locations where the geographic conditions were right. Long, low beaches protected from the tides are perfect locations to collect ocean brine and let the sun evaporate it away, leaving sea salt.

Both mining and making sea salt were expensive, so salt has been a valued commodity throughout most of human history. Many cities were founded near salt mines and wars have been fought over access to salt. Up until several hundred years ago, only the wealthy generally had access to salt in their diet. Even today, salt is not easily available everywhere and is not as heavily used as it is in the Western world. In some isolated populations in the Amazon region of Brazil, sodium intake is ten times lower than that in most industrialized countries.

Throughout history, the most common use of salt has been to preserve food rather than to flavor it. With the development of agriculture and animal husbandry, humans found they could feed, protect and raise a family living in one place. But the seasonality of growing crops and hunting meat required them to find ways to keep food in storage for months. It was discovered that items like meat, fish, vegetables, and even dairy products could be preserved by coating the surfaces with salt to make it last for the winter season or in times of famine. It's possible that humans thus developed the taste for salt as a byproduct of survival needs. Even modern day refrigeration has not taken away the desire for salt in our diets.

Does the Body Actually Need Salt?

The biochemistry of the human body indicates that we have a need for a small amount of salt in our diet, by which we mean the two chemical components of salt—sodium (Na) and chloride (Cl). It doesn't matter if the salt comes from rock salt mines or ocean brine, as both types are chemically the same (although sea salt may contain other minerals the body can use). Salt contributes to fluid balance, blood pressure, muscle activity, and the transmission of electrical signals.

At the cellular level, sodium controls water movement in and out of the cells. This is vital, for instance, in intestinal cells that are responsible for absorbing sugars from food and transforming them into the glucose the body needs. To help you better understand this, I will give you a brief overview of the biology and chemistry involved. You won't need any prior knowledge of either subject to follow this explanation, as it is accompanied by illustrations.

There are three natural sugars in foods. Both *sucrose* (natural fruit sugar) and *lactose* (milk sugar) are double sugar units, with sucrose containing one molecule each of glucose and fructose, and lactose containing one molecule each of glucose and galactose. The third sugar is from complex carbohydrates, which yield *maltose*, a double sugar unit containing two glucose molecules.

The digestion of complex carbohydrate begins in the mouth where the enzyme *amylase* secreted by salivary glands begins breaking the carbohydrate down. The activity of the amylase continues in the stomach until it is inactivated by stomach acid. All complex carbohydrates are digested into maltose within 30 minutes of leaving the stomach because of the action of amylase released by the pancreas. The stomach does not have the enzymes to break down sucrose and lactose so they enter the intestine intact.

Double sugar units cannot be absorbed into the body until they are separated into single sugar molecules. Cells that line the small intestine have enzymes that can split each double sugar unit into single sugars. However, double sugar units need to be in solution to enter the cells containing the enzymes. When the double sugars make contact with the outside of cells that line the intestine, sodium and chloride are both released, dragging water molecules with them. The water dissolves the double sugars, enabling them to flow into the cells of the intestinal wall, where each type of double sugar unit is split into single sugars. Sucrose is split into glucose and fructose, lactose into glucose and galactose, and maltose into two glucose molecules (figure 19).

In addition to helping dissolve the sugars; sodium activates transporter proteins, similar to the action of insulin, that facilitate the entry of glucose into intestinal cells. In fact, without sodium's help, no complex carbohydrate can be absorbed into the body. Although the pancreas has a duct through which digestive enzymes are released into the intestine, this channel is not used to release insulin to facilitate absorption of glucose from the intestine. The reason why sodium, not insulin, activates glucose transporters in the intestinal cells is because if insulin is released into the intestine it will be taken apart by the digestive enzymes.

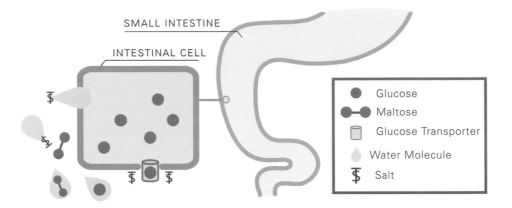

Figure 19. Salt drags water towards double sugar units. The water dissolves sugar which is broken into single sugars. Salt also activates glucose transporters. The body needs sodium to absorb glucose from the intestine.

The glucose molecules can now enter the bloodstream going to the liver where they can be either stored as glycogen, or released into the blood to be used by any cell in the body for energy, or converted into triglycerides for storage in the fat cells.

Galactose is transported in the same fashion from the intestine as that of glucose while fructose is transported by the random-facilitated method. Hence the rise in blood sugar level after the consumption of fruits is slower, as mentioned earlier.

The importance of sodium in this process is pivotal. Starting in infancy with the lactose in milk, the human body is programmed to absorb all the double sugar molecules passing through the intestine (unless the specific enzyme for splitting them is not working, such as in lactose-intolerant people). As we start eating solid foods, the increased intake of carbohydrates means that there are more double sugar units in the intestine and thus the need for more water to transport them to the cells of the intestine. This requires more sodium molecules in the body, not only to hold more water in the blood that can be sent to the intestine to dissolve double sugar units as they arrive, but also to help with the absorption of single sugar units into the body. The brain, in turn, causes you to desire more salt as it knows sodium is needed to manage the carbohydrate intake. This process is likely behind the fact that many people crave more salt in their diet as they eat more carbohydrate.

In addition, sodium ions also help transport glucose molecules in the kidney so they can be reabsorbed in the body before reaching the bladder, where they would have been urinated out. This process is probably an evolutionary adaptation to ensure that we do not waste any glucose.

The Problems Caused by Too Much Salt

While we do need some salt in our diet, it is equally clear that humans do not need very much. One proof of this is that there is no storage area in the body to keep salt. It is true that humans also have no storage area for water, but the two needs are not comparable. There is a vast difference in the amount of fresh water the body needs each day versus how much salt we need. The human body would need a significant appendage if we had to walk around storing our water, whereas only a small area to store salt might have evolved if we really needed a lot of sodium to survive.

Putting too much salt into your bloodstream creates the conditions for many problems. The first of these is the "sodium-carbohydrate" syndrome mentioned above. Consuming excessive amounts of carbohydrates prompts your brain to desire more sodium to handle the extra double sugar molecules that need to be broken down into glucose. This, in turn, causes you to desire more salty carbo hydrates, which launches you into a weight gain pattern.

A second problem has to do with the fact that sodium ions attach to water molecules. This causes your body to begin holding onto too much water, increasing the blood volume. A significant increase in the volume of blood results in the elevation of blood pressure. Those of you who have high blood sugar and high blood pressure would greatly benefit from reducing your intake of salt.

Our Natural Need for Salt is Going Haywire

Our taste for salt is a developed one. Infants do not crave salt. Newborn babies show an innate preference for a sweet taste rather than saltiness. In fact, if a child's carbohydrate intake is kept to a minimum, by about the age of four, it is unlikely that child will crave as much salt as a child whose diet has included a lot of complex carbohydrates.

Introducing complex carbohydrates with added salt into the diet of infants and consuming them repeatedly is the trigger that causes the body to start adapting to higher and higher levels of salt intake. It becomes a self-reinforcing cycle, as the increased intake of carbohydrates in one's daily diet creates an increased need for sodium to process the glucose, which in turn prompts us to eat even more foods with a high salt content or salty taste in order to obtain the extra sodium.

There is another brain regulatory factor that comes into play in causing salt cravings, and that is the generally high energy density of salty foods. Humans consume significantly more energy from foods classified as salty compared to foods classified as sweet (think bread versus cake to make a sandwich). In other words, your brain begins to make a strong correlation between salt and energy intake. In effect, the brain begins to adapt to a higher salt intake and enhances the signals it sends you to consume salty foods if they are high in energy. This is why both obese and non-obese subjects do not differ in their tolerance for the salt taste. Both types of bodies need energy, and salty foods taste equally pleasant to both. The only difference is that most obese people eat far more salty, high-energy carbohydrates than lean people, which is why they have become obese.

There is another factor involved in the spiraling cycle between more carbohydrates leading to more salt leading again to more carbohydrates. It has to do with the fact that as you consume more salt, your saliva increases in its sodium content as well. In order to taste sweetness, your taste receptor cells must interact with one of the natural sugars: lactose, maltose, or fructose. For the interaction to take place, nutrient molecules have to become associated with the receptor in the right configuration. However, a high concentration of salt in the mouth impedes the solubility and registration of sugar molecules with the sweet sensing taste receptors. In effect, this delays the taste sensation of feeling satisfied when you eat complex carbohydrates and so you end up eating more.

Studies confirm extremely high levels of salt consumption among children and adults today. According to the World Health Organization's review of sodium intake around the world, grain products contribute 38-40 percent of the sodium in the diets of children and young adults ages 4-18 years.[1] In 2007, the average American consumed 4000 milligrams of sodium daily compared to 2300 milligrams thirty years prior—that's an extra teaspoon of salt per day.

The body is able to handle a small increase in the amount of salt, but only up to a point. It does this by matching the salinity of the blood with that of the fluid around cells. If your salt intake makes your blood too saline, your brain will instruct you to become thirsty—the body's natural response to needing to lower your salinity. If you don't drink water soon enough, the brain can also instruct the kidneys, through hormones, to decrease the amount of water in the urine so more water is preserved in the body. Once you drink enough water, the kidney will excrete a large amount of it to remove the excess salt in the body. Thus, the body can accommodate increasing amounts of salt as long as, over the long term, you excrete almost precisely the same amount of sodium ingested.

How Much Salt Should Be In Your Diet?

The answer is very little. In general, your body does not need much of this nutrient. An adequate intake of salt is between 1200 and 1500 milligrams daily (not the 4000 mg you may be getting, as cited above). According to the American Medical Association, any food containing more than 480 milligrams of sodium per serving should be considered a high-salt food.

Rather than using a numeric standard, however, I have been suggesting that the best indicator of what and how much you eat should be determined by what your brain needs to obtain and maintain a level of nutrients necessary for normal bodily functions. If you start relying on your brain's regulatory system, you will naturally eat very little salt. If you were heeding the signals from your brain, you would know to stop ingesting salty foods just by using your taste buds and smell receptors. In effect, your taste and smell sensations tell your brain the nutrient concentration in your food, while your brain is comparing the current level of that nutrient in your body. Stated another way, if something tastes good to you, your brain is telling you that it contains nutrients you need. When a food

---

[1] *Sodium Intakes Around the World,* Elliot P and Brown I, October 2006, Paris ISBN 978-92-4159593-5

item stops tasting good, your brain is telling you it no longer needs any more of the nutrients in it.

In this way, evolution has made the sensations generated in response to the taste and smell of food valuable to us not only to identify and select what we should eat, but also to help us choose the most nutritional foods. When foods taste and smell good and have a pleasing temperature and texture (called "palatable" foods), we eat more of them. In one study, participants ate meals they rated high in palatability that were 44 percent larger than meals they rated low in palatability.[2]

There is, nevertheless, still a problem with the taste test for salt. As we mentioned, the body needs more and more salt to process higher levels of carbohydrate consumption. If you eat a lot of carbs, you will feel as if you need more salt. Furthermore, as you age, your body starts adapting to a higher intake of salt. This throws your brain's regulatory system off and you no longer have a biologically accurate method of assessing how much salt you should consume. Signals of taste generated by the saltiness of foods do not convey the same nutritional information to your brain as natural foods. This can make using the taste test for salt an ineffective way to judge when you have eaten enough of it. In fact, since your body may be craving more salt to help process the high amount of carbohydrates you are eating, you might end up eating even more salt.

Most people do not notice their increased tolerance for tasting salty foods because it occurs gradually. As mentioned, when we are infants we prefer sweet tastes; it is only as children consuming complex carbohydrates that we learn to tolerate, and eventually crave, the taste of salt. Over time, foods with a higher salt content begin to elicit a more pleasing taste sensation compared to lower salt versions of the same food. With experience, we learn to choose foods that contain a high salt content.

There are several other behavioral factors that contribute to a growing tolerance for salty foods.

- As your desire for salt increases, your body adapts to having more salt in your blood and cellular fluids. This means that your saliva is more salty.

---

[2] J.M Castro, et al, Palatability and intake relationships in free-living humans: characterization and independence of influence in North Americans. Physiology and Behavior 70 (2000) 343-350

When you eat, your taste cells are informing the brain about the nutrients in your mouth, so if your saliva is already salty, food will need to be a degree more salty for you to taste it. This causes you to believe you need higher and higher levels of salt just to taste your food and is why many adults add salt to their food to enhance its taste.

- The salt content of many prepared and canned foods is extremely high. Sometimes a single serving contains as much as 30, 40 and 50 percent of the entire Recommended Daily Allowance of sodium. Many people choose prepared and canned food products for convenience without considering the sodium content. Use of these products encourages higher salt intake.

- The food industry manufactures many food preparations, such as snack foods, with a mix of salt, sugar, and fat calculated to increase the taste and enhance the appeal to consumers. These foods have little nutritional value. The enjoyment of such foods can be intense and cause cravings for that food to develop.

- Condiments such as soy sauce, mustard, and tartar sauce are often used to enhance the flavor of a food item while masking its saltiness. Restaurant cuisine that uses these ingredients is generally high in salt, which further reinforces your taste for salty foods.

- When high salt food is consumed at a party or holiday gathering, it reinforces your enjoyment of such food. People often consume more salt-containing food in a social setting than when they are eating alone. For example, one study showed an increased intake of cookies when eating with friends than when eating with strangers.[3]

How to Start Controlling Your Salt Intake

It is possible to reduce your taste for salt. Studies have shown that individuals who gradually limit salt in their diets adapt to less salty foods and come to actually prefer these.[4]

---

[3] Clendenen VI et al. Social facilitation of eating among friends and strangers. Appetite 1994;23:1-13
[4] CA Blais, RM Pangborn, NO Borhani, MF Farrell, RJ Prineas, and B Laing. Effect of dietary sodium restriction on taste response to sodium chloride: a longitudinal study. Am J Clin Nutr 1986;44:232-243

Here are some recommendations.

1. Cut down your consumption of carbohydrates. We live in an environment where nearly every global cuisine has evolved to incorporate more and more complex carbohydrates into everyday meal preparations. The intake of complex carbohydrates has contributed to the largest share of food-related weight gain in the United States. Therefore, reducing your intake of carbohydrates is the most important action you can take to limit your body's need for salt. Evidence shows not only a reduction in blood sugar, but also in blood pressure (most likely from reduced salt intake) in individuals with Type 2 diabetes who did not consume whole-grain carbohydrate foods compared to those who consumed it.[5] A lower salt diet will, in turn, help you reduce your carbohydrate intake.

2. At your meals, stop eating when the food is no longer enjoyable to eat. This is your brain telling you that it no longer needs any of the nutrients left on the plate. To sense this moment of diminishing enjoyment, chew your food slowly and savor the tastes. You will find yourself becoming keenly aware of how highly salty many foods taste and will naturally lose your enjoyment for eating these foods.

3. When you cook, try gradually decreasing the amount of salt you add. Cut the salt you add to your dishes by 1/8, then 1/3, then ½, and finally to the lowest amount of salt possible so that you can experience the natural tastes of vegetables, meat, chicken, and fish. You will find that it is easy to begin appreciating the natural flavors and will eat less when you take the time to enjoy their taste. In cooking, use herbs and spices rather than salt to transition your brain back into being able to taste foods without salt.

4. Pay attention to the sodium content of foods when shopping. The "enjoyment of food" principle is key to helping you begin changing your shopping and dining habits to reduce your sodium intake. As you become aware of the overly salty taste of many foods you eat, you will stop purchasing foods that contain high levels of sodium. Follow this guideline: *Don't buy any food products*

---

[5] Jenkins et al. Effect of Legumes as Part of a Low Glycemic Index Diet on Glycemic Control and Cardiovascular Risk Factors in Type 2 Diabetes Mellitus. Arch Intern Med 2012;172(21):1653-1660

containing ingredients that could interfere with your taste buds' enjoyment of the natural nutrients. Here are some specific rules of thumb about shopping:

- At the grocery store, avoid items containing more than 480 mg of sodium in one serving. Rely on food labels to assess this because your taste buds may be unable to detect how salty some prepackaged foods are. Your saliva may already be so salty that your brain cannot accurately assess how much extra sodium is in a food item.
- Avoid buying processed foods marketed as ready-to-eat single servings because these foods are likely to contain high levels of salt and the serving sizes are determined by the manufacturer.
- If you buy canned vegetables and legumes, rinse them under cold running water. This can reduce their salt content by about 40 percent.
- Buy raw nuts that you roast without salt as snacks. Roasting walnuts without oil in the oven makes an excellent snack food.

Dealing with Salt and Carbs When Dining Out

Dining out at restaurants or as an invited guest in other people's homes is challenging when you are trying to change your eating habits, especially cutting carbohydrates and reducing your salt intake. Avoid going to restaurants that specialize in fried foods or cuisines that use a lot of fat, butter, and cream to disguise the saltiness. If you have some favorite restaurants that fit in this category, order items prepared as naturally as possible. If you have a favorite dish that is salty, eat only half of it and order a fresh salad on the side, then save the other half of the dish to eat at home or at work another day.

Changing your dining out habits can be challenging. The restaurants you patronize will remain as enticing as always. Dishes you enjoyed will look as attractive and smell as appetizing as before. You can still experience the pleasure your brain is expecting, but if you follow the advice here, your enjoyment will no longer be based on the volume consumed, but on the taste you extract from each bite. The end of the meal won't be determined by the emptiness of your plate but by your taste buds telling you they are no longer enjoying the food.

Similarly, if you are invited to a friend's home and presented with a dish made with a high salt, sugar, or high butter preparation, show appreciation to the host and chef by eating some of the dish but not a large helping. Remember that you do not need to equate your gratitude with how much food you consume. This can be difficult in some cultures where hosts not only feel insulted if guests do not eat everything on their plate, but encourage them to eat more than one serving.

Whether dining with other people or at someone's home, here's one strategy that you might try, not only to help yourself but to educate the people you love around you. Explain to your friends and family that you are eating using what you learned in this book about the nutrients our bodies need, the linkage between carbohydrates and salt, and the growing risks of diabetes affecting people in all walks of life. Perhaps your family and friends will feel motivated to change their eating patterns with you. If a movement to halt the pandemic of diabetes develops and the majority of people in this country begin altering their eating behavior, it will be an antidote to the food industry that keeps on producing unhealthy foods and to the restaurants that serve large portions of carbohydrates and salty foods.

KEY POINTS

- We have a need for a small amount of salt in our diet; it contributes to fluid balance, blood pressure, muscle activity, and the transmission of electrical signals.

- Consuming excessive amounts of carbohydrates prompts your brain to desire more sodium to help with absorption into the body from the intestine and reabsorption from the kidney.

- Beware of the fact that, if we continue eating a high carbohydrate diet as we age, we increase our tolerance for salt and the chance of developing diabetes.

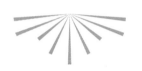

PART 4

Eat What You

Enjoy & Enjoy

What You Eat

To eat is a necessity,
but to eat intelligently is an art.

—FRANÇOIS DE LA ROCHEFOUCAULD

CHAPTER 25

A Complete Overhaul in How You Eat

You have learned about the real cause of high blood sugar leading to diabetes. You have learned how the brain monitors your nutrient intake and guides you in determining what and how much to eat. The previous chapters have also covered weight gain and rediscovering your authentic weight, as well as the role carbohydrates play in contributing to excessively high glucose levels in your blood. You have learned how to break out of the salt-carbohydrate syndrome. Finally, you now know why and how you need to cut out carbohydrates as the main source of triglycerides that are filling your fat cells, causing the switch to burning fatty acids rather than glucose in your muscle cells.

Part 4 is aimed at my fourth revolutionary idea regarding a whole new approach to eating, which I have termed "conscious eating." The foundation for this approach is based on reconnecting with the vital signals that your brain gives you about hunger and satiation based on its ability to measure your nutrient intake and usage. Your brain has the same remarkable capability of monitoring your hunger and taking inventory of your nutrient intake as it does of monitoring every element of your life. Just as your brain can evaluate your surroundings and warn you of danger, or listen closely to a symphony and pick out the piccolo part, or feel an itch in your lower back when you are giving a speech to an audience, it can detect the nutrient needs of every cell in your body and assess whether you need food.

To listen to and respect your brain's signals about hunger and satiation, you must learn to reject the other mechanisms by which you make decisions about when and what to eat. Many of these patterns of behavior are supported by scientists who believe that satisfaction during a meal is more psychological than it is physiological. They view satisfaction as happening when the person stops eating, and since this is earlier than the time needed for digestion to complete and does not depend on calorie content, they suggest it is a psychological decision, not a physiological one. Such scientists subscribe to sensory adaptation and habituation as the psychological component of satisfaction. This refers to the many unconscious rationales that have formed into patterns of behavior based on your family's habits, your culture, and your personal psychology, which have taken over your brain's nutritional regulatory system.

But the fact is, there is a natural physiological mechanism based on taste and smell signals starting in infancy that you can apply to regulate your food intake, even as adults. Nature has provided you with the ability to accomplish the task of meeting your daily nutrient needs. Picture yourself as a toddler. Your brain prompted the sensation of hunger whenever you needed nutrients. It told you to stop eating when you consumed enough of the available food. This same knowledge is stored in your memory and you can go back and retrieve it.

The question is how, as an adult, do you retrain your mind to make use of your natural human mechanism that regulates food intake? How do you create the desire and motivation to return to using these birthright mechanisms that are already in your brain to regulate food intake?

The following chapters will show you. A clear understanding of the mechanism behind the generation of the hunger sensation before a meal and the satisfaction signal during the meal will allow you to recognize when you actually need to eat and why you don't need to engage in overeating, leading to weight gain. I will also teach you a new approach to conscious eating that involves relearning how to eat for enjoyment—chewing your food slowly and fully, allowing the nutrients to register in your brain, while paying attention to your body's signals that you have eaten enough and have satisfied your nutritional needs.

These chapters will help you develop the new thought patterns you need to achieve your goal or return to your authentic weight. The motivation for these new thought patterns should not be the fear of developing Type 2 diabetes or its complications, but rather your confidence in your ability to reactivate the nutrient regulatory mechanism you used for many years during your childhood. If you have the desire to take charge of your weight maintenance and avoid high blood sugar and diabetes, you can do it.

KEY POINTS

- To listen to and respect your brain's signals about hunger and satiation, you must learn to reject the other mechanisms by which you make decisions about when and what to eat.

- If you have the desire to take charge of your weight maintenance and avoid high blood sugar and diabetes, it takes new thought patterns that you can learn to create.

After implementing what Dr. Poothullil recommends, I lost thirty pounds. In fact, I seem to have trouble gaining even a couple of pounds back when trying to, as instructed by my family doctor who wanted me to have "a little reserve."

Nelson, Overweight Adult, Oregon

CHAPTER 26

Why Do We Get Hungry?

Some people wake up in the morning and feel immediately hungry for eggs, toast, pancakes, or cereal. Others have no appetite for several hours; a glass of juice and a coffee out the door are sufficient. Later in the morning, you might feel the need for a little snack—yogurt, a muffin, or perhaps carrots and celery if you are trying to eat more fiber.

At some point mid-day, most people begin feeling definite pangs of hunger—a craving that can be fulfilled only with a hearty sandwich, a bowl of soup, or even a full luncheon plate of meat, chicken, or fish and vegetables. Towards mid-afternoon, your stomach may call out to you for an energy infusion to get you through the rest of the day. Then at dinner time, depending on your eating habits, you may indulge in a small meal to complement the nutrition you had so far during the day, or perhaps a very large meal that finally satisfies your desire to eat plenty and well. Later in the evening, you may find yourself dreaming of a sweet—and so you raid the fridge or freezer for one more item.

These are the patterns of eating in the US and in many Western societies—three meals per day of varying sizes, plus morning and afternoon snacks, and perhaps an evening dessert. If you were not reading this book, you might continue eating this exact way for the rest of your life, following the same routines you learned in childhood, which are reinforced by our highly scheduled culture organized around work hours and school for kids and adopted by millions of families throughout the industrialized world.

The question is, do you need all this nutrition? Are you actually listening to your brain's hunger signals? Do you know what your hunger signals are and how to respond to them properly so you do not over-consume energy nutrients your body does not need?

This chapter explores the nature of hunger and how your brain communicates to you when, what, and how much you should eat.

What Causes Our Hunger Sensation?

The sensation of hunger can be more intense than any other human feeling or desire. What causes the brain to generate this sensation? After all, the body is programmed to store a certain amount of fat that you can use to draw energy from rather than continuously eating every day.

Since fat is created and taken apart on a continuous basis, could the total quantity of fat falling below a certain threshold level be responsible for the brain generating the sensation of hunger? Probably not because if this were so, your sensation of hunger should stop once your fat stores are above a certain level and not resume until they fall below the threshold. For example, if you gained one pound of fat in the past week, shouldn't you stop feeling hunger until that fat is used up? Conversely, if you lost several pounds of fat in a month, why don't you eat continuously until that fat store is replenished to the threshold level? Both of these do not happen.

Let's test another explanation: Could the sensation of hunger occur when the level of fat circulating in your body (in the bloodstream and fluids around cells) has gotten too low? But this too is unlikely because the amount of circulating fat is small compared to the total fat in the body. Stored fat quickly converts to fatty acids which can be reconstituted by the liver into circulating fat. So there should be no need to eat simply to increase the amount of fat circulating in the body.

A third explanation for hunger might be that our low fat stores release a messenger of some type to notify the brain that we need more nutrition. The fat cells actually do secrete a small protein called *leptin* which has been identified as a potential messenger candidate. However, nothing about leptin molecules in their amount, structure, or function has been linked to causing the hunger sensation to be generated in most individuals.

A fourth possible cause of hunger relates to the glucose reserve in the body, which is limited to less than about 120 grams of glycogen in the liver and about the same in muscles. These stores can be rapidly depleted during the period between meals. Therefore, might the hunger sensation be signaling the brain that we need to restore the glucose reserve in the body?

Again, this is unlikely. If low blood sugar is the cause of the hunger sensation, then why do people with diabetes feel hunger even when their blood sugar level is far higher than normal? One might argue that diabetics have a lower level of glucose inside their cells or that their sugar metabolism is defective, so they cannot be representative of the general population. However, even people who do not have diabetes feel the sensation of hunger when their blood sugar level is artificially kept high using a glucose drip into the vein.

Could the hunger sensation be generated by the arrival in the brain of a hormone released by the stomach or another part of the gastrointestinal tract? Ghrelin, a hormone released by cells in the stomach, can increase the intensity of hunger. But to date no one has identified a hormone that *initiates* the sensation of hunger or even a mechanism that activates the release of this hormone.

None of these explanations appear adequate or correct. As discussed before, I suggest that the answer relates to the brain's nutritional regulatory system. The brain has an enormous capability of tracking the level of nutrients in our body, right down to the cellular level. The power of the brain to monitor and track our nutritional needs is no less extraordinary than the capacity of the brain to recall an incident that happened to you 30 or 40 years ago, to tell the muscles in your hand how to coordinate with your eye to play ping pong, or to recall the words and phonetics that allow you to speak a language.

Given this, I contend that the hunger sensation is generated when the brain detects a critical level of depletion not just of glucose but of key nutrients essential for the normal functioning of the cells of your body. This is why even diabetics with high blood sugar feel hunger. The brain, being the command center of our nutritional regulatory system, knows when many key nutrients will soon be lacking in addition to glucose. Just as the brain detects an insufficiency of water in cells and bodily fluids and generates the sensation of thirst, it signals hunger when it detects that other needed nutrients are about to fall below optimum levels. This explains why you can feel the sensation of hunger at unpredictable intervals of time, even within a short time after eating if not enough of some nutrient has been consumed (figure 20).

Your Brain Determines Your Selection of Foods

If the above is true, one might wonder how the brain knows what foods it needs when it sends out the signal for hunger. After all, when you are hungry, you usually have a wide choice of items to choose from whether you are at home, at your office, or on the road. If it seems that we randomly choose what to eat based on what is in the pantry, what restaurants are nearby, or who we are with, how do we manage to get the nutrients that our brain has identified as lacking?

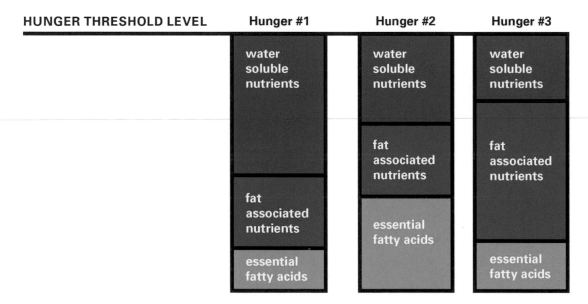

Figure 20. Your brain detects what and when nutrients are lacking. The deficiency of each nutrient is added up to a threshold level. This is why the hunger sensation can be experienced at any time, not just at fixed intervals during the day.

The answer is, your brain does attempt to guide you towards the right foods either through the unconscious decisions you make about what to eat or via conscious cravings you have for specific foods. The brain has learned and knows which foods can provide you with the missing nutrients. It has correlated the information stored in memory of foods you have already eaten and their nutrient components. These correlations began forming at the beginning of your life and continue to be made on an ongoing basis, building a database of nutrient-food correspondences that the brain uses to guide you.

In effect, the brain's regulatory system tracks your food and fluid intake during each meal and compares it, when possible, to the nutrients received from past experiences with the same foods. Your brain knows what nutritional value you get from a hamburger, a spaghetti dinner, wonton soup, a burrito, chicken curry, or whatever foods are in your cultural background. This capability of the brain is no different than how a toddler can listen to the same story or music over and over and the child's brain learns the words so that he or she can complete the story or song when listening to it later. In the same way, your brain becomes a databank of foods and their nutritional values—and pushes you to desire certain edibles when you need their nutrients. Consider all those times when you find yourself asking, "What should I have for dinner tonight?" and an answer pops into your head without any trouble. That is your brain telling you what nutrients it needs.

These messages are different for each person, of course, reflecting their past eating experiences, culture, and food preferences. The brain guides each of us first towards foods from which it knows it can obtain the necessary nutrients. For instance, onions, garlic, rice and curry are meaningful sources of nutrients for some people and their brain will desire foods containing them. For others, these items will seem unpleasant to their brain, which prefers meat, salad, and potatoes because it knows their nutritional value.

Of course, this doesn't mean that people do not eat and enjoy new foods. That said, for most of history, humans have had very limited choices of food. In many ways, having access to so many foods offering an enormous variety of nutrients, is an evolutionary leap. Each time we try a new food item or recipe, the brain updates its database, adding the new item and the nutrients it supplies to its inventory. This is why it's easy to enjoy foods from other cultures and begin craving them as much as foods you grew up with when you feel hungry.

When you start a meal in response to the hunger sensation, your brain has already determined the need for nutrients. Your taste and smell receptors begin to immediately track the foods you consume and relay to the brain the type and amount of nutrients they contain that will soon replenish what the body needs. This reinforces the importance of chewing slowly and thoroughly to release as many nutrients as possible for detection.

Your saliva contains enzymes capable of converting carbohydrates and fat into smaller molecules that are sampled by taste and smell receptors during your meal. From the number of times the taste and smell receptors are stimulated by a nutrient and from the knowledge stored in memory as to the concentration of the nutrient in the food being consumed, the control center calculates the quantity of nutrient likely to be swallowed up to that point.

However, the mere registration by taste and smell receptors is insufficient for the brain to produce a sense of satisfaction related to the intake of any one nutrient. Otherwise, the strong smell of a nutrient needed only in a minute quantity or just a taste of that nutrient could cause the control center to produce the sense of satisfaction without your having consumed enough of it. This is why, for instance, when your body needs vitamin C, it is unlikely you will feel satisfied after drinking just a single sip of orange juice. If your body needs iron, your brain knows that a mere taste of red meat is not enough.

Instead, the brain waits to determine its satisfaction when the first swallows of food or drink arrive in the intestine and signals are sent out to confirm the nutrients. This allows the brain to make a better measure of the signals generated by the taste and smell receptors regarding which nutrients are in the food items and how much of each are entering the body. After you swallow several times, the brain can more reliably conclude, from the combined registration of nutrients by the taste buds and in the intestine, which nutrients will soon enter the bloodstream. One proof of this are animal studies showing that if the food taken by mouth is allowed to drain out through a hole in the stomach, with no food reaching the intestine, the animal will eat for a longer period of time than normal because the intestine is not registering the arrival of nutrients.

This is not to say that you completely restore all your nutrient deficiencies in any one meal. Some necessary nutrients may not be available in that meal. Also, the body is constantly changing in its needs. This is why even when you feel satisfied with one type of food on your plate, other foods not yet eaten can still seem appealing because they have other nutrients needed by the body. You may be willing to stop eating the meat while wanting more of the broccoli or the potatoes.

After each meal, the brain seeks to correct any unmet needs in subsequent meals. Signals related to the nutrients needed but not yet obtained are likely added to the signals of other nutrients that are now becoming scarce in the body. With adequate nutrient reserves in the body, however, the brain can wait several hours for complete absorption of nutrients from one meal before reassessing what more you need—and regenerating the sensation of hunger again. However, this means you have to rely on multiple meals of varying sizes to get all the needed nutrients on any given day.

You might wonder why people with very high levels of sugar, fat, and cholesterol already in their blood feel hunger. Again, this could be understood by the fact that the body needs many nutrients for normal functioning. Hunger is the only sensation the body can generate to make sure that you consume all needed nutrients. In other words, the brain appears to have a natural inclination to acquire any nutrients the body needs, even when it has an excess of other nutrients and even if eating results in consuming nutrients you do not immediately need. It is also possible for people, as they get older, to become conditioned to eat at certain times of the day, whether they are hungry or not, just as they prefer a certain combination of foods during breakfast, or drink a particular beverage with their meals.

The biology of digestion and nutrient absorption is far from being completely understood. But my view is that the brain's signals to us about hunger and its attempt to steer us towards certain foods could be linked to the fact that the body needs to be able to utilize all available nutrients and this requires many nutrients and agents around to absorb, transport, and break them down. It is likely that there are many interactions between nutrients that we are not yet aware of. Further study of nutrient interaction is needed.

Significance of the Nutritional Sensory Regulatory Concept

This explanation of why we get hungry is consistent with a regulatory mechanism of nutrient intake based on our sensory experiences. It is applicable to humans of all ages—infants, toddlers, children and adults. It clarifies how your smell receptors initiate salivation to start the digestion process even before a morsel of food enters your mouth, or how they trigger rejection of food that could be detrimental to your health. Your sensory experiences in the taste buds of your mouth send messages to your brain, which stimulates the release of insulin into the blood to prepare for the nutrients that will soon be released by the intestine.

Your nutritional regulatory system is no different than how your other senses prompt your brain to react to stimuli. For example, while looking at a painting, your brain appreciates colors of varying intensity and the lines of demarcation between them. When listening to music, your brain can differentiate the rhythm, loudness, and tempo of notes from different sources of instruments. This in-the-moment enjoyment of the painting and music is possible because signals travel to and between neurons in the brain at speeds faster than 250 mph (which is a very fast speed considering the small space inside our heads).

In the very same way, the brain acts as a regulatory system that uses the senses to determine the nutritional value of what we eat. As toddlers, we would not be able to develop an appetite for foods without a natural mechanism to monitor the nutrient needs in the body. Toddlers would also be unable to consume adequate amounts of foods for normal growth and development without a natural mechanism to measure incoming nutrients and assess how much is needed and what is missing.

I am encouraging you to let your brain do its work of matching the intake of nutrients that pass through your mouth to the deficit in your cells that it has already identified. When you pay attention to your food during a meal, your brain will recognize nutrients by the signals generated by your taste and smell sensors. If you are preoccupied with some other thought or action, your brain may not be focusing on recognizing the nutrients being consumed. Paying close attention to your meal allows the brain to record and react to the nutrients passing through the mouth. Taste and smell sensors are ideally located to assist your brain in accomplishing the tasks of monitoring nutrients in your body and metering new ones entering it.

All you have to do is to become more aware of the intensity of your enjoyment when you eat, as this is your brain's pleasure signals that you need the nutrients. It's natural to enjoy eating, but the key to regulating your food intake is to completely enjoy what you eat by focusing on the sensations you experience when you taste the food. Try paying attention to these sensations the next time you sit down for a meal and you will begin to detect a noticeable difference in how you approach eating.

The fact is, hunger enhances the intensity of your enjoyment. When you start your meal in a state of hunger, chances are your body needs multiple nutrients. Some may be needed only in minute quantities and others in larger amounts. When you are hungry, your brain creates a greater intensity of response to each bite of food, which you experience as enjoyment, based on the signals coming from your mouth, taste buds, and smell receptors. The amount of time your senses come into contact with nutrient molecules is much more important in experiencing enjoyment than the quantity passing through the mouth.

Being able to enjoy your food requires that you keep your taste and smell receptors healthy. Nature does its part by replacing taste cells every few days. Nerve cells that detect smell sensation are replaced at the rate of one percent each day. It is your duty to keep these sensors in proper working order through oral hygiene, including brushing and flossing your teeth. It is important to stay hydrated as well to ensure you have a good salivary flow.

In summary, when you get hungry, eat healthy and enjoy what you eat to the maximum.

KEY POINTS

- The brain guides us first towards foods from which it knows it can obtain the necessary nutrients.

- Paying close attention to the intensity of enjoyment your brain derives from your meal allows you to better determine your level of satiation. The amount of time your taste and smell senses come into contact with nutrient molecules is much more important than the quantity passing through the mouth.

- You do not completely restore all your nutrient deficiencies in one meal. After eating, the brain seeks to correct unmet needs in subsequent meals.

CHAPTER 27

How Your Brain Signals You to Stop Eating

We just explored the hunger sensation—what it is, why you become hungry and how your brain guides you into fulfilling your hunger through the selection of foods you eat and the brain's ability to track your nutrient intake. Now let's look at how your brain provides signals to stop eating. In effect, both hunger and satisfaction are determined in the brain.

In general, the brain abides by three principles that govern the generation of satisfaction. The first is whether you have acquired the needed nutrients in sufficient quantities. The second is whether you have relieved the sensation of hunger. And the third is how it can prevent you from overeating.

To accomplish these goals, the brain generates the feeling of satisfaction and fullness using four types of signals sent through your blood circulation and via the intestine, stomach and mouth. Like hunger, these signals of satisfaction are generated subconsciously and automatically. Like hunger, these signals are highly dependent on your body's nutritional status. At some meals, you may need multiple nutrients and can eat a large quantity of food until your brain recognizes that you have consumed all the nutrients necessary. At other meals, your brain will be quickly satiated after you have eaten only a small amount either because you needed only a small number of nutrients, or the available food did not have any of the needed nutrients, or it could reflect the fact that the food you consumed was very rich in the needed nutrients.

Signals from the Mouth

Your mouth plays a significant role not only in the enjoyment of eating, but also in giving you clues to stop eating. These two parts are associated. The enjoyment of eating starts with the mouth feel of the bite of food you just took. I'd like to stress that the tactile experience of eating comes from the texture of the food and not from the feeling of fullness in the mouth from a single large bite of food. Textures of foods differ. You'll find yourself chewing each bite of some foods multiple times, which will add to the tactile experience.

But how can chewing help the acquisition of needed nutrients, relieve the hunger sensation, and prevent overeating? First, the act of chewing and grinding breaks food into smaller particles and even molecules, which helps the brain begin to measure the amount of nutrients you consume. Second, the movement of your lower teeth by the jaw muscles also registers inside your brain and adds to the tactile experience of eating. If you were to have blended or pureed food pumped directly into your stomach through a tube, not only would you dislike what you are consuming, you would have trouble deciding how much to take in to feel satisfied. On the other hand, if you are allowed to chew the food before putting it through the tube, you would not only enjoy what you are consuming, but also would feel satisfied with less food compared to the amount put through a tube without your chewing it, even though you did not actually swallow what you were eating.

The key principle here is to heighten your awareness of the sensory experience and the mechanical actions *combined.* Both of these are critical. By paying attention to the sensations created in the mouth during the act of chewing, the brain has an open channel of communication to inform you what to do next: continue eating or stop eating via the quality of the sensory experiences generated by your taste sensors and smell receptors. As you eat and start to fill yourself, the combinations of signals from these sensors and receptors cause your brain to respond by creating a drop in the intensity of flavor of the food. This deliberate act by the brain helps regulate your food intake. When you stop enjoying what you eat, you will put down your fork.

Signals from the Stomach

The volume capacity of the stomach is a second source of signals to limit your intake during a meal. As food descends through your esophagus into the stomach, it forms concentric circles in the body of the stomach. The first mouthfuls of food lie along the inside of the stomach wall and form a layer as newly swallowed food accumulates on top of it. The stomach normally has relatively little tone in its muscular wall, allowing it to expand and bulge progressively outward.

Relying on the feeling of fullness to stop eating is like relying on the feeling of the fullness of a water balloon to determine when to stop putting in water. Because the balloon can stretch, you can put a lot of water in it before it gets full—a point which is almost impossible to know beforehand. Similarly, your stomach muscle can keep stretching to accommodate a large quantity of food—up to more than one liter in volume—before you feel full. Recall how you can feel full by the end of a sumptuous meal, but still eat dessert. You're able to do this because your stomach expands.

At some point, the stomach relays the sensation of being physically full to the brain. The problem is, when you feel that full sensation varies depending on the tone of your stomach muscles.

Signals from the Intestine

From the stomach, food next enters the small intestine, where hormones are released. Some of these hormones reach the brain center in charge of food intake through the blood, informing it that nutrients in the intestine will soon be absorbed. After receiving this confirmation, the brain begins to reduce the intensity of hunger you felt. Similar to how your car triggers a sensor in the street causing the light to change from red to green at the intersection, the signal from your intestines to the brain causes you to slow down your eating. The sense of satisfaction your brain has from the hormone signal is not based on the quantity of food you have eaten, but on the arrival of nutrients. It can be useful to remember that fat-containing foods such as nuts speed the release of intestinal hormones faster than carbohydrate-based foods, so your hunger abates more quickly. If you are hungry for a snack, it is better to eat nuts rather than carbs such as chips.

You can test your brain's response to intestinal hormones in the following way. Next time you are hungry, put the amount of food you normally have on a plate and eat slowly for about ten minutes. When you have eaten two-thirds of what is on your plate, walk away and leave the remaining food behind. Drink some water to cleanse your mouth. You may still feel the urge to eat, but within about ten minutes, the intestinal signal will reach your brain. It will now be about twenty minutes after you began eating and you will find that your desire to eat more has diminished markedly. Your sense of feeling satisfied will be close to what it would have been if you had finished the whole meal.

Signals from the Blood

After the digestion of food in the intestine begins, nutrients such as glucose are released and absorbed, causing glucose levels to elevate in the bloodstream. The blood circulating in the brain now knows that you have responded to the feeling of hunger, and starvation has been averted. This further prompts the brain to produce a sense of satisfaction and well-being. This signal takes about 30 minutes to register after you start eating and many hours to complete from the time you began the meal.

Paying Attention to the Multiple Ways to Stop Eating

Why do we need so many different ways to stop eating? The human body needs multiple mechanisms because many internal and external circumstances can affect what and how we eat. The body may need to override the signals from the taste sensors and smell receptors if the brain detects that not enough nutrients are being consumed. Similarly, the brain may sense that not enough of the nutrients available in smaller quantities have been digested in the intestine and signal you to keep eating, even if this means you may be overeating other nutrients you have already consumed. For example, if you have ever eaten a light lunch of a plain green salad, you may have found that you continued to feel hungry. This is because your brain required the nutrients found in proteins from legumes, fish, or meat.

From a survival point of view, this biological backup system of four types of signals would appear to be better than one system based on eating enough of a certain nutrient. If your brain informed you to terminate eating the moment you had enough of just one or a few of the nutrients needed, you might never fulfill your body's need to consume many other nutrients. The overeating of some nutrients in one meal is usually rebalanced by eating less during later meals.

It makes sense that the brain's priority is to enable the body to consume the maximum number of needed nutrients from the available food at each meal. Therefore, the brain makes it possible for you to enjoy more food, even after eating to satisfaction, regardless of the method used to terminate the meal.

KEY POINT

- As you eat, the combinations of signals from smell sensors and taste receptors cause your brain to respond by creating a drop in the intensity of flavor of the food. This is when you should stop eating, regardless of the availability of more food.

Through Dr. Poothullil's help and putting into practice the ideas in EAT CHEW LIVE, I have lost over 100 pounds. It has given me hope that there is another way to care for diabetes, think about food, and eat.

Randy, Type 2 Diabetic, Texas

CHAPTER 28

Three Reasons People Overeat

You probably love food. It's hard to resist a good meal. But until you began reading this book, you may not have thought much about food as a collection of molecules containing the nutrients your cells need to function. You of course know that food provides your body with energy and vitamins and minerals, but what has been missing in your understanding is the impact of what you eat at the micro-level, where food breaks down into single molecules of energy nutrients and essential nutrients. You probably also never thought about your brain as a regulatory system that actually monitors and tracks your nutrient intake—using your taste sensors, smell receptors, the sensations in your mouth, the hormones in your stomach and intestines, and the levels of glucose and nutrients in your blood as it flows through the brain.

If these sophisticated mechanisms have developed in humans, why do we overeat? Why doesn't the brain help us completely regulate our sensations of hunger and satisfaction such that we never gain weight, never consume too much food that floods our bloodstream with glucose, and never develop high blood sugar and diabetes?

I suggest there are three reasons why people override their brain's regulatory system and overeat:

1. Dopamine based: eating for the pure enjoyment of eating even when not hungry.
2. Fullness based: eating only when hungry, but continuing until feeling full.
3. Stress induced: eating to relieve stress and anxiety.

People who tend to overeat often do so for two or three of these reasons rather than just one. The commonality between these is that they all demonstrate that when we overeat, we override the brain's hunger and satisfaction signals.

Let's examine these three reasons to better understand them. In the next chapter, we will discuss how to overcome them.

Dopamine based: Eating for Enjoyment without Being Hungry

The factors that fuel the desire to eat when you are not hungry are likely complex. As an infant, toddler, and very young child, you probably did not overeat when you were not hungry. Most very young children tend to be completely in touch with their hunger and satisfaction signals. They only eat when hunger drives them to do so and then only as much as they can handle.

I suggest that non-hunger eating begins more or less as a temporary and occasional accident, done without recognizing its long-range significance. In most people, it occurs as incidental to other events or situations, such as a family picnic or holiday dinner, a chance meeting with a friend, or an unplanned spur-of-the-moment meal with someone. It is not a deliberate act of eating, but a random occurrence.

However, the more these eating events occur in one's early life, the more repetition reinforces the brain to make connections between eating and enjoyment. Whether you are hungry or not, if food is available and appealing, you learn to feel it is okay to eat it. You may sense that it's not appropriate to be eating when you are not hungry, and even those who cared for you during your childhood might have told you not to do it. But little by little, you begin to rationalize that since food serves a good purpose, eating just a little bit without being hungry can't be that bad. The enjoyment of discovering new foods and the pleasure of eating them eventually overcomes your natural inclination to wait for the sensation of hunger.

Over the years, your mind develops ways to rationalize and minimize the unwanted consequences of this eating behavior. You may start to gain weight, but tell yourself, "It's just a few extra pounds and I can take it off easily." You may know that you are eating too much, but dismiss it by thinking, "I can stop doing this any time I want, but for now, I'm enjoying this food." This pattern of eating may even be strengthened by those around you who are doing it, too.

A repetitive act is reinforced when it is accompanied by strong feelings. In this case, it is the pleasure associated with food. You begin to establish a behavior of eating when stimulated by the sight, smell, or even just the thought of food rather than by your body's hunger signals, just because you like the feeling of enjoyment. The connection between food and enjoyment is stored in your memory and expresses itself without any conscious or deliberate effort. Smelling food cooking, walking into a colorful supermarket, passing by a restaurant—all these trigger in you a pleasurable feeling caused by the release of *dopamine*, a neurohormone, that prompts you to want food. You look forward to enjoying a variety of good quality, tasty foods.

Once this rationale is established, however, you may easily fall prey to craving foods that combine sugars, salts, and fats of different properties in optimum ratios to create items that intensify the feeling of pleasure you seek.

Once you reach this stage, even your awareness or the presence of adverse long-term consequences such as weight gain, high blood sugar, high blood cholesterol, or high blood pressure may not be sufficient deterrents to modify your response to food. This is because the brain has difficulty connecting behavior with long-term consequences. If the ill effects do not immediately follow the causal action, it is easy to rationalize a behavior. Your subconscious mind can't make value judgments, deciding whether what you're doing is good or bad. It simply remembers and accepts what you have been doing and facilitates the execution of the established behavior. The behavior continues, even when the consequences are damaging.

This pattern of behavior is not unlike other behaviors you might cultivate for pleasure, such as gambling, work, sex, or even accumulating wealth. Once you begin the activity, it becomes difficult to stop repeating it over and over.

Fullness based: Eating Only When You Are Hungry . . . but Overeating

If you are good at waiting for your hunger signals and not eating prematurely when your body needs nutrition, what would cause you to be unaware of the signals of satisfaction your body generates for you? There are likely several possible explanations for this behavior.

The first might be that you overeat in the sense that you simply consume too much of the wrong food. Your diet may emphasize grain-based carbohydrate, natural sugars, salt, and fat that provide your body with an excess of nutrients it cannot immediately use. While you may believe you are eating appropriate portions, the fact that your choice of foods is skewed means you are filling your body with glucose, fatty acids, and salt. The more you eat these foods, the harder it becomes to maintain your authentic weight and to prevent the onset of high blood sugar and possibly diabetes.

This type of overeating can also begin unconsciously. While hunger triggers the conscious decision to initiate eating, your subconscious mind is not controlled by rational thought and is easily swayed to follow eating patterns you established long ago. For example, if as a child or teen you repeatedly consumed fruit juice or soda in response to thirst, the subconscious mind can interpret the thirst sensation as a need for soda and not water. (Are you one of those people who drink soda all day long?) If you routinely had eggs and bacon for breakfast when you grew up, the brain could create a craving for these in the morning even though the body does not need nutrients from these items. In effect, you may be hungry when you eat, but you consume too much of the wrong nutrients out of habit.

The second reason you may overeat is similar to that of a person who enjoys food and has built up a behavior based around the pleasure of eating. You may wait for the hunger signal, but once it starts, your enjoyment takes over and you cannot stop yourself. However, instead of variety or quality, the quantity of food becomes the pleasure-generating factor for you. You have long stopped paying attention to the feeling of satisfaction during a meal. You wait for the stomach to stretch almost to the point of discomfort to stop eating.

Your uncontrolled enjoyment may also have started accidentally by overeating at family events, parties, business outings, and trips to new places where abundant (and sometimes free) foods are found. Repeated overeating at such events reinforces the feelings of pleasure you derive from getting full, and they become ingrained in your unconscious mind. The absence of immediate negative consequences following an excessive intake of food can lead to a behavior pattern in which you rationalize overeating with excuses such as, "I was really hungry" or "I just wanted to taste that new dish," or "I skipped lunch so it's okay if I eat a lot at this party." You might also be influenced to consume a lot of food by external factors such as dining with friends who overeat, going to an expensive restaurant where you want to partake of the luxury and get your money's worth, and many other situations.

Stress induced: Overeating in Response to Stress

Stress is any stimulus that alters the meaning or intensity of your feelings, actions, or communications. Signals that you interpret as harmful to your safety, security, or wellbeing are the ones that cause a stress response. The stimuli that cause stress are essentially the same for most people—perceived threats, illness, injury, overwork, unsolved work issues, family problems, relationship issues, or inconveniences. The intensity and duration of the stimuli needed to elicit the stress response varies for each person. One individual may be able to handle many difficult life events that another person would find highly stressful. It seems true that one's conditioning and training to cope with stress starting in early childhood and continuing to adulthood determines your sensitivity to stressful stimuli.

In general, people experience stress as two powerful feelings: fear or hurt. Fear can be imagined or real and based on known or unforeseen factors. Fear, by definition, is more emotional than rational. During the fear response, neurons located in the primitive core part of the brain are activated before the stimulus can be analyzed on the intellectual level to determine if it is real and deserves a thoughtful reaction. Fear rather forces you to determine what to do based on an incomplete analysis of partial information. Hurt can be physical or emotional. It can be based on a current event or a past experience.

The time of onset, degree, and duration of the stress response vary with each individual, based on hormones released in the body during the stress response. For instance, let's look at anger, a feeling of displeasure aroused by a real or imagined stress. If your body releases adrenaline at the slightest provocation, you're a person who will get angry quickly and easily. If the amount of adrenaline released is large or if your sensitivity to it is high, the intensity of your anger will also be high. If you remain in the stressful environment or dwell on the stress in your mind, your body can continue releasing the hormone for a long period, setting the stage for prolonged anger. If you routinely expect a person or event to create displeasure for you, it may cause you to be angry each time you encounter that person or event.

How and why does stress cause people to overeat? The two are actually quite connected. As you recall from earlier discussion, adrenaline is released in the body in between meals to facilitate use of fatty acids as fuel. If you become stressed when you're hungry, or vice versa, more adrenaline is released. One of the reasons eating helps you feel better is because food in your digestive system helps slow the release of adrenaline. The experience of feeling calmer and more relaxed after eating sets up a behavior pattern that promotes eating when you feel stressed.

A second reason people eat when feeling stressed is that the body's stress response causes you to seek out some action to mitigate the stressor. You feel you have to do something to relieve the stress. For many people, the action of preparing and eating helps them stop thinking about the stressor or believe that they are managing it. Through the repetition of this behavior, eating often becomes an automatic process for stressed-out people to meet the challenges of their lives.

The irony about stress is that some people enjoy creating a sense of stress out of ordinary life events because they become habituated to the adrenaline in their body. They heighten events through thoughts that make them feel internally stressed, out of which they believe they become more energetic. In their mind, stress sharpens their focus and helps them perform at a higher level. They actually feel lethargic without some stress in their life. Some utilize stress in a creative way to accomplish their artistic objectives. Others may invent a stressful situation just to experience a thrill. For example, those who drive at high speeds or ride roller coasters do so for the pleasure they get from putting themselves in stressful situations.

Some "adrenaline junkies" use food or drink to counteract or complement their love of stress. They may drink coffee, soda, and sweetened beverages frequently during the day. In their jobs, they may drive themselves to keep working right through lunch time, scarfing down snacks and carbohydrate-rich foods and guzzling soda to hold them over until dinner time. In the evening, with their body depleted of energy, their brain is hungering for good nutrition so they finally eat a full meal. However, their lack of balance and control during the day often drives them to overeat as this becomes the only opportunity they have to enjoy their food— and so they overindulge in the pleasure of eating. This again becomes a common behavior pattern for stress junkies.

How Your Brain Reinforces the Pleasure of Eating

We need to recognize that the apparent innocuous "over-enjoyment" of food is a common theme among all three types who overeat. In all cases, we saw how random and accidental instances of overeating might initiate a seemingly innocent habit that you are initially able to find excuses for. But with increasing repetition, the rationale you give yourself for overeating becomes embedded in your subconscious mind. Little by little, overeating is transformed into a consistent behavior pattern of adulthood. It doesn't matter whether you overeat when you are hungry, not hungry, or under stress. Overeating becomes part of your conscious behavior. You believe you can consume as much as you want, even in the presence of side effects that you dismiss.

When the instinct to eat is repeatedly supplemented by a habitual inclination to overeat and eventually replaced by it, your brain has activated the area that generates a desire to eat while suppressing other areas that usually warn you about the dangers of overeating. You have replaced your instinctive pattern of eating for nutrition because you now have a different priority—*deriving pleasure from eating.*

At the core of this behavior is the "pleasure mechanism" in the brain that controls the nutritional regulatory system. This mechanism utilizes two complementary sets of neurohormones. The first set that the brain releases to create satisfying feelings are *endorphins*, which are morphine-like neuropeptides released in the brain. These are the brain's natural painkillers that produce a sense of well-being and calm. This neurohormone may have originated as a reward when the body met basic necessities such as nutrients.

As mentioned above, the second neurohormone is *dopamine*, which produces the feeling of pleasure when you imagine a good meal. The dopamine system may have evolved as a way to feel rewarded by meeting the body's need at times of extreme deprivation of water, salt, glucose, and other nutrients. This feeling can be more intense than endorphin-based satisfaction because the situation was dire. For example, when feeling extremely thirsty, drinking a glass of water can be one of the most pleasurable feelings you have.

From a biological standpoint, the human body was not constructed to overeat on a consistent basis and gain excess weight to the point of causing high blood sugar and diabetes. As stated before, the body doesn't need to store more than a small amount of fat. The purpose of our digestive system and fat cells are to capture nutrients we might need on an immediate "just-in-time" basis. Similarly, the brain's neurohormone system of endorphins and dopamine was designed to produce feelings of satisfaction and pleasure when we consumed food that supplied our body with the nutrients it needed. The neurohormone system complemented our hunger and satisfaction signals.

What is happening to humans in much of the world is exposure to an endless variety of foods that activate our excitement and pleasure. It is biologically natural to feel a desire to eat these foods. But as we begin eating too much of the wrong foods that are mass produced in our industrial food complex—grain-based carbohydrates, natural sugars, fats, and salt—we reinforce behaviors that repeatedly trigger the pleasure system of the brain. We thus begin overeating regularly because it induces these pleasurable feelings and we are no longer content to feel the enjoyment that comes with eating enough to feel just satisfied.

Evidence of this abounds in Western societies where high blood sugar and diabetes are rapidly increasing. Restaurants continue to serve extremely large portions compared to the amount of food a normal human actually needs for nutrition in a single meal. Some restaurants even make an entire business out of offering people expansive 'all you can eat' specials, as if to challenge them to overeat until they are bloated and sick. Sugared drinks and food products packed with carbohydrates and salt are packaged and marketed in ways to make us associate them with happiness, sexuality, success, and good times. Even when people cook at home, they have trained themselves through habit to serve large portions and eat everything on their plate regardless of the signals they may receive from their mouth.

The occasional and random overeating that might have happened when we are young becomes a routine and acceptable lifestyle for most adults, driving an inevitable pandemic of high blood sugar and diabetes. I am not denying that food is enjoyable and creates pleasurable feelings in the brain. However, whether you overeat when you are hungry, not hungry, or stressed out, you lose control of your brain's two natural systems—the nutritional regulatory system and the pleasure system. This is unfortunate, because heeding these systems could prevent you from falling ill and possibly dying early.

People in Western societies are losing control of the natural human mechanisms to eat healthy and enjoy their food to powerful external forces that are motivated by profit—the food industry and marketers of food products. Diabetes has existed as a rare human condition for thousands of years, a biological phenomenon based on bodily chemistry. However, with obesity in some countries now reaching 30 to 35 percent of the entire population and being seen in children as young as ten years old, and diabetes affecting an estimated one-third of the entire global population, it is clear that factors outside of normal human biological phenomena are driving epidemic levels of this disease. Nothing short of a revolutionary approach can reverse this epidemic.

KEY POINTS

- The three reasons why people override their brain's regulatory system and overeat include eating for pure enjoyment even when not hungry; eating only when hungry but overeating, and eating to relieve stress and anxiety.

- Non-hunger eating often begins as a temporary and occasional accident, but through repetition, the brain connects overeating and enjoyment.

- The "over-enjoyment" of food may seem innocuous at first, but through repetition, it becomes a habit and you replace your instinctive need to eat with *deriving pleasure from eating,* despite negative consequences for your body.

CHAPTER 29

How to Modify Your Eating Behaviors

Is it possible to gain control of your eating behaviors, specifically at those times when you cannot stop yourself from overeating in one of the three ways just described? Fortunately, the answer is yes.

Some readers may be thinking, "Of course, it's easy to stop myself from overeating. I could do it anytime I want to." If that's true, then why haven't you done it yet? If you are overweight or have been diagnosed as prediabetic or diabetic, you have not yet understood on a deep level how to control your eating behaviors. This chapter will teach you how to achieve this control.

Many of you might be thinking the opposite, "I simply can't stop myself from indulging. I love food way too much and I can't figure out how to stop overeating. I don't see how I can change my habits." You may feel skeptical of trying another approach if you have experienced failures with other "lifestyle changing" attempts.

Whatever your reaction, I want to help you feel confident that you can regain control of your overeating habits. If you begin to reflect on what you have learned so far in this book—the real cause of high blood sugar, the serious impact that eating a high grain-based and salt diet creates, and how your brain's nutritional regulatory system can help you listen closely to its signals of hunger and satisfaction—you can make meaningful changes in how you eat. This chapter will show you how.

How the Brain Forms Patterns of Behavior

Your mind is ultimately responsible for your behavior. Each behavior you have consists of an input that triggers it, nerve impulses through the brain that process it, and an output that manifests itself in your actions. Your brain receives information internally from each and every organ and system in your body about its working conditions, needs, and threats. It also receives information from your external senses—taste, smell, touch, vision, and hearing.

All these inputs generate electrical, molecular, or heat-related signals that are transmitted to the brain not in their original form, but as nerve impulses, which are pulses of electricity. Your sight is converted into nerve impulses, pain in your finger is converted into nerve impulses and your thinking about an ice cream cone is converted into nerve impulses.

Neurons throughout different parts of your brain respond to these signals by generating their own electricity. Every brain cell is composed of three parts: the main body, the peripheral nerve or axon and tiny projections from the body called dendrites. The contact points between neurons lie on the surface of the dendrites and the body. Signals are transmitted through the gap called a synapse between the contact points. Each synapse can have over 100,000 channels for transmitting signals from one neuron to another.

The resulting electrical field pattern in the brain defines your state of mind at any given time and your resulting actions. For example, even a simple activity like throwing a baseball generates thousands of signals to the brain from the skin, muscles, tendons, and joints. The fingers of the hand holding the ball generate signals indicating the type of grip and the feel of the ball's leather surface, firmness, warmth, or coldness. When you throw the ball, your eyes generate more signals about its location and trajectory, the height the ball reaches, how far it went and where it landed. If another person is playing catch with you, even more signals are sent to the brain. Meanwhile, internal signals created in the brain determine your purpose and the execution of your action.

If we think of the brain as a sort of computer, then the nerve cells are your hardware and the patterns formed by your life experiences are your software. The software is programmed when brain cells respond to the input of information from any source and make connections to other specific brain cells.

Chemicals called neurotransmitters released by one neuron stimulate receptors on another neuron through selected communication channels. The type and amount of chemicals released in the synapse and the duration of their stay there determine the nature of the information transmitted, or not transmitted, from one neuron to another. Neurotransmitters allow the transmission of electrical impulses only in one direction. This one-way conduction makes it possible for the brain to direct transmission toward specific areas of the body.

Each set of connections that the brain develops between neurons in response to various internal and external stimuli and neurochemicals around the neurons constitute a sort of program. The input your brain receives and the information that is already stored in it determine your actions and communications. As these signals travel through the brain, a mental picture is formed with the help of different sets of neurons residing in multiple areas of the brain. Information on the "what," "where," "when" and "why" of each event is stored in multiple sites in the brain and maintained by permanent changes in connections and neurons.

The speed with which connections between nerve cells are made is the highest during the first few years of life, when each brain cell gets connected to thousands of other neurons, forming all the programs that help you through life. One program allows you to pick up a fork, another to write, another to think about a poem, and so on.

How the Brain Loves One-Way Thinking

The above information is significant when it comes to understanding how to change any behavior. This is because the brain effectively works by forming very stable patterns of "neuron networks." The linkages formed between neurons involved in all your software programs are like crisscrossing strings of Christmas lights that share some of the lights. When your senses stimulate any neuron in one string, it can light up the entire string linked to it. But some of the same neurons in a string may be involved in more than one network. With individual neurons responsible for specific pieces of information such as time, place, or people, they serve as common links between different experiences. When the information entering the brain relates to a time, place, or persons you already know, the brain tries to make associations with strings existing in memory containing the same time, place, or persons. Of the multiple strings established, many are strengthened and retained but some get blocked or are eliminated due to lack of use.

Over time, your brain's nervous system becomes organized into highly functioning groups of local networks, each handling different thought processes or tasks. When the brain detects a familiar pattern during processing, it directs the electrical impulses through one of these pre-established channels, using a one-way traffic system with stop signs. As you repeat a behavior, the signal path for that behavior becomes automatic. Once a pattern of response is established

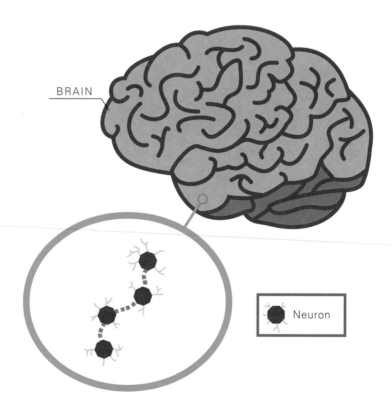

BRAIN

Neuron

Figure 21. Over time your brain's neurons become organized into highly functioning groups of local networks, each handling a different thought process or task.

through repetition, or if the experience has an emotional significance, it becomes etched in memory. Thereafter, the same incoming stimulus produces the same response with only minimal processing (figure 21).

There are good reasons that the brain operates in this fashion to establish specific networks and adhere to signal transmission through clearly established pathways. Foremost of these is the absolute need in the brain for order, without which it would be unable to function. Most of the neural connections formed in a human embryo are related to the functions of vital organs needed for survival. Without strict adherence to clear transmission channels, the brain centers that control vital functions such as heartbeat and respiration would be unable to perform their activities properly and life itself would come to an end.

For example, if your survival is threatened and your body needs to activate muscles to escape, your muscles need more fuel to generate needed energy. This involves increasing the heart rate to deliver the fuel. In addition, to convert the fuel into energy, more oxygen is needed. The centers that control heartbeat and breathing need to send and receive signals to and from the appropriate organs in an instant. Similarly, when you exercise, the brain must make quick adjustments to your body to maintain normal metabolic operations. As part of its automatic response, it alerts the heart to beat faster, the lungs to breathe faster and deeper and the skin to begin sweating. It is the brain's automatic responses *through established pathways* that allow these types of responses to occur immediately. Since these functions are needed throughout one's life, it makes sense that transmission pathways need to be as secure and permanent as possible (figure 22).

Another reason the brain establishes and strictly adheres to specific signal pathways is to protect all brain centers from stray electrical impulses intended for some other area of the brain. Since each neuron has the potential to respond to many incoming stimuli, proper safeguards are necessary to prevent neurons from responding to signals that other specialized networks need to handle. For example, if a network of neurons is already trained to regulate heartbeat, then unnecessary signals reaching them could cause irregularities in cardiac function.

A third reason the brain forms specific networks is to conserve energy through faster action. A person expends a lot of mental energy learning a new activity, but after the person practices that activity for several weeks their brain uses much less. Experiments show that the processing period for perception

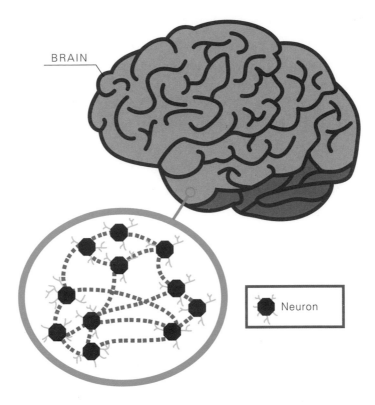

BRAIN

Neuron

Figure 22. Inside the brain, neurons link up into millions of crisscrossing networks (pathways). These ensure rapid response to stimuli, protect brain centers from stray electrical impulses intended for some other area of the brain, and conserve energy through faster action.

becomes less with training. By choosing a pre-formed pathway, the brain saves both time and energy that it would have spent testing multiple pathways and then selecting the best one during each input.

For example, recall when you were learning to drive and how new the various actions were to your brain and muscles. You had to learn how to brake just right—not too hard, but not too soft—when approaching a red light. This required understanding and feeling how your car behaves when you push the brake pedal down, as well as learning to judge the distance between your car and the stopping point, how speed and road conditions impact braking and how to hold the steering wheel steady when stopping. If you had not mastered all this, imagine how taxing it would be to drive all the time. If you've ever driven in a snow storm, you know how energy draining it is because you cannot rely on your usual auto-pilot driving skills, but rather must rely on your senses and muscles to ensure safe driving.

A fourth reason the brain depends on automatic pathways is to be able to multitask, a necessary element for survival. Imagine that you're attentively listening to an important conversation. While the conscious mind is processing the incoming voice inputs, the subconscious mind is processing noises from the surroundings through established pathways. Any change in the loudness or timbre of the external noises might force the subconscious mind to alert the conscious mind to pay attention so that you can decide whether there is a threat to your survival requiring immediate action or if it can be safely ignored.

Finally, pre-formed pathways make learning more effective and efficient because gaining any skill or knowledge requires your brain to access memories of what you already know. The biological basis for learning may come from our innate survival mechanism. By having established behavior patterns for what we have already learned, we can more easily distinguish new events from what's familiar. The brain dislikes the uncertainty of new experiences. This is why we feel tense when we get into circumstances we don't know or understand. The brain immediately senses it has to learn something new to cope with the unknown, and that it has to form new pathways.

Given the brain's natural inclination to form and adhere to specific neural pathways, it makes sense that it resists any attempt to change a single neural pathway. The brain conducts thousands of activities simultaneously to inhibit and modulate any undesirable actions and seeks to protect these patterns. Modifying a neural pathway is a threat because if the brain's usual inhibitory control is modified, unwanted desires can emerge. For example, during sleep, when the brain's inhibitory controls are not in full force, you may have dreams in which you take part in activities that you would not consider doing if you were awake. In addition, if established pathways could be easily altered, it might be possible to overwrite even newly formed pathways, making it difficult to establish a reliable behavior pattern.

How to Break Old Patterns to Change Your Eating Behavior

Throughout your life, each time you have eaten something, your brain has received millions of signals from your taste and smell receptors. Each experience has produced specific connections between nerve cells in your brain to form a pathway about eating, which has itself been strengthened through repeated use. The way you have been eating has effectively been 'hardwired' and solidified as a neural network in your brain. It has become self-sustaining and, more importantly, hard to change because it's not stored as a file that can easily be deleted.

It used to be thought that once the brain had established most of its connections during childhood, it only changed in response to aging. However, it has come to light that the brain has the ability to rewire itself to form new connections with different neurons to create groups of neurons that can learn different solutions to obtain a different result. This resourcefulness of the brain can be used to overcome an established behavior and accomplish a positive outcome.

When you learn something, new nerve connections are established and consolidated. Unlearning requires weakening of the established connections between neurons. Because this work has to be done piecemeal, it takes time. However, the brain has natural mechanisms that can help you learn a new behavior while unlearning an old one. Interestingly, nature has provided a hormone called *oxytocin* in the brain to dissolve existing connections so that new ones can be formed. Without this process, the brain could become saturated with old pathways with no room for new connections, new networks, or new behaviors to form.

Luckily, the adult brain is reasonably accustomed to unlearning. If you ever moved homes or changed cities to study or work in a new city, you probably had to change your routines and habits. If you started living with someone, you had to rearrange millions of brain pathways to accommodate that person. Such unlearning requires "de-connecting" established neural paths and making new ones, one pathway after another and one network of neurons after another. The point is, somewhere in your past, you have unlearned some things and learned new ones. You can do it again. The same unlearning and new learning called "neuroplasticity" can help to retrain yourself about how and what you eat.

To establish a new behavior pattern that promotes healthy eating, begin by finding ways to restrict activating the established pathways that promote unhealthy eating. Here are some recommendations to begin unlearning by unraveling established pathways you have about food:

- Walk around your home and identify the areas and sights that test and break your control over food—and eliminate or modify them. For example, put all food in cabinets where it can't be seen.
- Don't shop for groceries on an empty stomach. Buy food only using a prepared shopping list so you are not tempted to buy extra items on impulse.
- Pre-plan your meals and portion sizes.
- Avoid locations that you associate with eating such as food aisles in convenience stores, fast-food restaurants, stores serving free food samples, and vending machines that prompt you to buy food on impulse.
- Work on creating an environment that is not focused around food in your home. If you are surrounded by pleasing sensations that are commonly paired with eating, it's hard to deny the impulse to indulge. The sight and smell of sweets like ice cream, cookies, and cakes can stimulate the urge to eat, so don't bake desserts and don't stock ice cream in your freezer. The goal is to decrease temptation by reducing the sights, sounds, and smells of pleasing impulses.

Tapping Into Your Willpower

You need to create a different way to initiate and complete food intake to begin forming new patterns about your eating behavior. Each action you perform in your life, including thinking about eating, requires the participation of thousands of nerve cells in the brain. When you start any action, those cells are already set to interpret signals in the way they have been programmed to do in your past. Changing your eating behavior, such as why you eat, what you eat, and more importantly how you eat, requires reprogramming nerve cells involved in the act.

In other words, you must relearn how to talk to yourself about eating. You may not have much control over the occurrence of sight, sound, smell and random thought-related cues that trigger your desire to eat, especially in places beyond your own environment. But you can moderate the effect of these cues by changing the processing that happens in your brain after these sensory impulses are received. For this, your brain has to decide consciously to override your old conditioned response. You have to be able to tell yourself that the smell or sight of food does not mean you must eat it.

We commonly call the ability to resist something "willpower." You need willpower to resist eating when you're not hungry and only eat when you are. To generate the willpower, you have to practice control over your impulse to eat. It is easier if you are already behaving in a disciplined way in other fields in your life. Most everyone has willpower in something in their life they can tap into. If you get to your job every morning on time, you likely have willpower that you can apply to your eating behavior. If you clean your house every Saturday without fail, you have willpower. If you take a shower every day, you have willpower.

Your thoughts are the manifestation of your will. Thoughts can be the results of your will to act or they can direct the will to form. It requires effort and training to keep your focus on beneficial thoughts. The good news is that an established thought process regarding eating can be modified based on reasoning driven by two important motivations. The first is this. If you train yourself to eat better, you can avoid a lifetime of medications to lower sugar and fat levels, unwanted side effects of the medications, and the unavoidable suffering from the complications of diabetes. The second is knowing that you will feel and look better and enjoy life far more by maintaining your authentic weight. Be aware that if your mind is preoccupied with thoughts of other pressing matters or inert with no sense of purpose, you may not feel the urgency to exercise your willpower.

Creating a Plan to Change Your Habit of Eating From Stress

It also helps to have a detailed plan for dealing with situations that cause you to eat out of stress when you're not hungry. If your eating behavior is governed by stress, you may need to adjust your response to stressful events in general before you can change your pattern of eating. This is because your eating response is interconnected with your reactions to stress, and thus runs through the many well-established and linked pathways in your brain. You may need professional help to create new pathways to deal with stress-related events, but here are some suggestions to start:

Stop thinking about stressful events. One way to reduce the impact of stress in your life is to minimize the amount of time you spend thinking about or discussing stressful events that don't personally concern you. If somebody is talking to you about their problems, feel sympathy, empathize with the person, and even show compassion by helping that person, but avoid getting emotionally involved in their predicament.

Don't project outcomes of your illnesses. If you have an injury or illness, reduce the stress of the experience by not allowing your imagination to run wild about an outcome that has yet to occur. It's easy to assume that you might have the same complications experienced by other people you have known with a similar injury or illness, but this anticipatory stress is unnecessary because it may not happen to you. Even if complications occur, they may not be as severe as you imagined.

Don't project outcomes of events. Limit your expectations about the consequences of events in your life to strictly what you have full knowledge of. Otherwise, developing feelings related to an undefined event outcome could become progressively more depressing, filling your mind with worry and affecting your bodily functions such as sleep. It doesn't matter if the stress is generated by an action or communication that impacts you negatively, or by the lack of an expected action or communication that should have benefitted you positively. Just try not to think about it repeatedly because each time you do, your brain not only recruits more neurons but also solidifies the connections between them, intensifying your stress.

Don't stress out over events that you will never experience, such as your own death. In order to answer the question how well you slept, you have to be aware that you slept by being awake to answer the question. In the same way, when you're dying, your awareness is diminishing. Once you're dead, you won't know that you're dead. You can't experience death and therefore shouldn't be stressed about it.

Learn to meditate. Yet another way to reduce the impact of stress is to establish a new string of neurons that deal with no signals by learning meditation.

One of the reasons meditation seems difficult is precisely because brain neurons by nature are programmed to respond to signals from outside the body, from internal parts of the body, and from other neurons. Meditation asks that you learn to quiet the mind by stopping all signal processing. Meditation is useful for people learning to retrain their responses because meditation can create a group of neurons that avoid all incoming signals, thus creating an environment of peace and calm. Escaping to this string of neurons during meditation allows those neurons that have been dealing with the stressful event time to rest, recuperate, and perhaps process the stress response from a new perspective using other sets of neurons.

Exercise. As mentioned earlier, adrenaline is released during a stress response. If some adrenaline can be channeled to promote another activity, the intensity of your response to stress could be proportionately less. The best way to accomplish this is to engage in a physical activity such as exercise. If you enjoy the activity, it may release hormones such as endorphin that can further reduce the impact of stress.

Rediscover the Eating Behavior of Your Childhood

I wrote earlier that most childhood eating habits are based on true hunger and satisfaction. You ate enough to grow and function but you did not overeat. Over time, however, your parents, the other people in your life, the environment in which you lived, the choices presented to you and your life experiences have all contributed to modifying your childhood eating behavior patterns. Your mission to rediscover and maintain your authentic weight may get a psychological boost if you think of your journey as reestablishing the eating behavior of your childhood so that it matches your body's need for nutrients. This image can help you internalize the feeling that if your need for nutrients is not real, you should not be eating. If the need is minimal, ask yourself if you can wait until your brain evaluates the need relative to nutrients in storage and then generates the sensation of hunger.

I realize this is very difficult to do. In the modern world, advertising directly and indirectly involving food often creates the urge to eat. Your exquisitely trained brain, instead of responding to nutrient needs, is tempted many times per hour to imagine the pleasure of eating. How does this happen?

You need to look deeply at what causes you to give into temptation. It could be that you just wanted to enjoy the taste out of curiosity. In other cases, the motivation could lie deeper than that, such as boredom from having nothing else meaningful to do, feeling unwell, or being tired. If stress is a frequent trigger for you to eat, you have to consider the possibility that in order to feel the enjoyment of eating, your brain is actually facilitating a stressful mood in you by creating drama in your life.

Every day, you must make decisions about what to eat. When you eat out or eat at somebody's house, you have less choice about what to eat because you're eating off a menu or what the host has cooked. You have to be alert when you decide to eat, choose the food you want to eat, and be aware during your meal to enjoy what you eat.

Just as a story is presented using groupings of different words, a behavior is formed by a series of nerve connections. To change the story line you need to dismantle multiple parts, if not the whole, of the original word groupings and form different ones. Similarly, to change your behavior you will have to destroy many established nerve connections and form new ones. This will take time.

The strength of your brain's existing networks is why it's easy to reactivate old connections and fall back into your former patterns. How much importance you give to the new way of eating will determine how effective you are at rewiring your brain. You must not only learn to do things that work, but avoid falling back into previous behavior patterns that promote excess consumption.

Imagine that an orchestra has been performing a variety of pieces. Now imagine that the musicians are asked to learn and perform a new piece which is very similar to another piece they have been performing, but with minor variations in note strength and the order of instrument participation. At the same time, they are asked to be ready to perform the original score. It would be hard for most of the members of the orchestra to avoid falling back to the way they were accustomed to playing before the variations were introduced unless they really concentrate.

There are times when you will find it hard to stick to your commitment. One common instance of this is when the neurochemicals needed for exercising self-control are not available. For example, at the end of a long day at work, it is possible your neurons may be depleted of the neurochemicals needed to generate a disciplined behavior. If that is the case, you could decide to postpone taking complete control and settle for a temporary state by eating a little bit of food even without the hunger sensation being triggered.

Once you begin making a few major changes to modify the neural networks in your brain and delete old connections, you will be able to establish new pathways for a different behavior around eating within several weeks. But making the behavior permanent may require months of practice. Repetition not only strengthens the connections between certain populations of neurons, but makes it easier to activate them. If you reach a plateau in your progress, it's often a sign that the brain needs time to consolidate the changes already made before further ones can be accommodated.

Establishing a behavior pattern conducive to maintaining your authentic weight requires commitment and determination, but once the pattern is firmly established it becomes relatively easy to follow. By repeating your new behavior day after day, changes in your brain connections will become more refined and the new behavior more automatic.

KEY POINTS

- Your brain contains many groups of neuron networks that have formed to quickly respond to stimuli. Your current patterns of eating are ingrained in these networks. This makes changing behaviors difficult, but unlearning can be done.

- To establish a new behavior pattern that promotes healthy eating, find ways to stop activating the established pathways that promote unhealthy eating.

- It may take several weeks to modify the neural networks in your brain and delete old connections about eating, but it can be done. If you reach a plateau in your progress, your brain needs time to consolidate the changes already made, so be patient.

CHAPTER 30

Eating Slowly
and Consciously

Eating slowly and consciously are perhaps the ultimate keys to health. Choosing the right foods and appreciating the nutrition in them are analogous to appreciating the colors and shapes that make a painting visually appealing. Feeling the mix of nutrients in your mouth is like listening closely to sound waves of different duration, speed, and grouping that hit your eardrum in an orderly sequence and make music pleasing. Nutrients are the elements that trigger the wonderful signals used by your brain to create your sense of enjoyment during a meal. Nutrients enter your mouth as a mixture of unpredictable variety and concentration in each item of food. Eating slowly allows more time for the generation of their signals to reach your brain.

You will be amazed, as you pass age 40, how little food you need during any given meal to sustain yourself until the next meal, unless your job requires strenuous physical activity. But while you need less food, you still require the same quality and diversity of nutrients as you did when you were younger. Since no one else but you can know your nutrient needs, you have to rely on your own internal monitoring and metering mechanisms to ensure you consume adequate amount of nutrients during meals. This means your ability to assess the nutrition in your food is directly proportional to the amount of time nutrients remain in contact with your taste and smell receptors. The more time you keep nutrients in contact with them, the more signals your brain receives—and the more enjoyment of food you have. In short, reducing the quantity of food you consume need not translate into the reduced pleasure of eating.

Your mission during a meal should be to eat what you enjoy and, more importantly, to enjoy what you eat.

The primary objective of this book has been to help you learn to stop eating any item of food when your body does not need the actual nutrition from it. You can assess this by listening closely to your brain's hunger and satisfaction signals. You can tell that you no longer need to eat the food on your plate as soon as the intensity of your pleasure in eating it diminishes. By paying attention to your natural control mechanisms to stop eating and by making an effort to change your past learned behavior to eat just to feel full, you can begin to empty your fat cells, lose weight if necessary, and begin living a healthy, diabetes-free life.

Let me make an analogy for eating consciously and slowly. Imagine yourself among a group of people scattered inside a closed 10 by 10 feet room. Someone releases a fragrance into the room from a concealed canister. Within seconds, you know the nature and concentration of the fragrance regardless of your location in the room. A few molecules of the perfume extracted from the air you breathe in are enough for your brain to know the properties of the perfume. Similarly, the association of only several molecules with taste and smell receptors is all that is needed for your brain to appreciate the nutrients being swallowed. Put another way, you swallow a lot of food without really enjoying it. This chapter will show you how to become a conscious eater, enjoying more of what you eat while reducing the intake of food that is not enjoyed.

How You Developed Fast Eating Patterns

If you reflect on your life, I'm sure you will admit that most of the time, you don't eat slowly. In our fast-paced lives, we tend to eat very quickly. Working people often gulp down their breakfast and lunch, either while driving or sitting at a desk at work. Even family dinner times may be hectic as parents are pressured to get the meal on the table after returning home from work so the children can have time to do homework or other activities. In my experience, most people don't spend sufficient time to truly savor the food, chew it slowly, and pay attention to their body's signals.

Eating fast is not a natural human way to eat. If you look at infants sucking on the breast or at a bottle, they usually go slowly, starting and stopping several times during a feeding. The physical contact with the mother and the availability of milk reassure and please the baby. When infants are introduced to solid food, they begin sensing the various flavors and tastes on their taste buds and smell receptors. They start establishing their food preferences. Eating habits, attitudes, and unconscious feelings about foods are created at this stage. In most countries, these are influenced by the culture, as food choices and flavors are passed from generation to generation and strengthened by association with rituals. But no matter what culture they grow up in, most children still eat slowly. The classic admonition from parents around the world is telling their child to, "Hurry up and finish your plate."

For adults, the changeover to eating fast occurs for different reasons at different times. You may have started rushing through meals during your early teen years so that you could do homework or run outside to play with friends. You may have started eating fast in high school or college so that you could spend more time with friends or a boyfriend or girlfriend. Or it might have begun when you started working in a job and found yourself under pressure to devote your lunch hour (or just 30 minutes for many people) to work rather than to enjoying your food.

Little by little, most adults begin adapting to eating faster, paying less and less attention to their choice of food and their body's reactions to it. They cave in to work schedules that allow little time to eat. Lack of time and the pressure to get things done often force them to take larger bites in order to quickly finish a meal. The same factors also cause them to speed up the rate of chewing and swallowing, which is why we call it "gobbling down" their food. With busy families, many adults often eat lunch or dinner alone with little impetus to "dine" and enjoy a slow meal while talking. Fast food restaurants become part of many adults' weekly routine—and the term "fast" applies not only to how quickly they receive their food but how speedily they consume it.

Another consequence of eating fast is that it changes your sensitivity to your body's signals to stop eating. In your younger days, you were apt to respond more often to the sensory signals coming from your mouth. When your brain decided that you had gained enough nutrients from consuming an item of food to meet the needs of your body, you responded by stopping the consumption of that food. As you got older, though, you may have started using signals other than those coming from your mouth to terminate the act of eating. If you frequently ate food without enjoying it and without paying attention to it, you began to lose touch with knowing when to stop. Over time, you trained your brain to prompt you to stop eating only when your stomach finally felt full, if not bloated. This increasingly became an automatic response during mealtime for you, even though you may have known full well that you were eating too much.

All these habits have reorganized your brain's former connections about food and established new ones that reinforced efficiency, speed, and the practicality of eating over the enjoyment of food and the pleasure of nourishing your body. Today, whenever you eat too fast to really enjoy what you are eating, whenever you clean your plate just to finish your meal (or get to the dessert faster), and whenever you indulge in food without being hungry, you continue to reinforce these neural connections and transform them into the only pathway that comes into your brain from eating. As a result, you become increasingly unaware of the high levels of carbohydrate, fat, salt, and sugar content of the foods you are consuming because you simply are not taking the time to taste them.

How to Eat Slowly

The act of eating slowly consists of three different stages.

- First, you experience the qualities of the food in your mouth by taking the time to chew it.
- Second, you decide whether or not the food is appealing before, during and after chewing.
- Third, you swallow the food.

Repeat this process with each bite until you're done with your meal.

The best way to train yourself in this new way of eating is to start with the act of chewing. During a typical meal, you take a number of bites. You chew each bite of food many times before swallowing. The more aware you are of the motions involved in chewing, the more you'll fully experience and enjoy the food before it disappears down your throat. You should be deliberate in chewing, feeling the force of each chewing motion. This will allow you to concentrate on the sensations generated during chewing.

Your goal is to literally taste every bite of food as it enters your mouth. When you chew it with the conscious intention of experiencing its nutrients on your taste and smell receptors, it completely changes the experience of eating versus simply biting into food, smashing it for a second or two with your teeth, then swallowing it within seconds. Chewing slowly fully breaks up the food, creating new surfaces from which flavor-producing nutrients can be liberated. Enzymes that are secreted by the salivary gland aid this process.

Some food is mixed with an enzyme called *ptyalin*, which breaks up complex carbohydrates, releasing the sugar called maltose. Sweet-sensing receptors on the tongue cannot detect the complex carbohydrates themselves, only the maltose released in chewing. Less than 5 percent of all the complex carbohydrates that are eaten will be affected by ptyalin. However, enough maltose can be released in the oral cavity for it to register with your sweet-sensing taste receptors and that is what your brain will enjoy.

Another enzyme called *lipase* breaks up fat, releasing molecules. Agitation and warming of the food during chewing allows fat-associated nutrients to waft up the back of the throat and stimulate the smell receptors, which need to detect only several of the molecules in each bite to register the odors and create enjoyment. If you savor cooked or barbecued chicken, beef, or fish by chewing it slowly, you will notice that your nose becomes increasingly sensitive to the odors, contributing to your pleasure of eating these foods.

Appreciating the combination of sensations from the textures, temperature, and flavor or "heat" from spices and the smell signals in your nose creates the full experience of each bite of food during a meal. Reliance on your taste and smell receptors to enjoy the quality and to determine the quantity of food consumed shows that you are in charge of your body.

Swallowing food without enjoying the flavor of it is like flushing a delicious dish down the drain without tasting it. Only when food is properly chewed can you receive the full palette of its tastes, flavors, and sensations. Proteins in general and meats in particular require more chewing compared to carbohydrates and cooked vegetables.

Here are some additional tips to help you learn to eat slowly and chew fully.

- When you take small bites you can better appreciate even the smallest amount of food you consume. Therefore, adjust the bite size of your food. The food should fit within the boundary of your teeth. When the mouth is closed, there is normally approximately a half-inch of space between the tongue and the roof. If the bite size is bigger than this space, the food has to be parked temporarily outside the boundary of the teeth or immediately swallowed. If you have to keep part of the food in your cheek, you have taken too big a bite.
- Always put food on your tongue when you introduce it into your mouth. Feel the texture of the food before you start chewing. This lets you enjoy the food from the moment you put it in your mouth, as enjoyment starts with awareness.
- During a meal, use your tongue to move food around the mouth, rotating it with your tongue. This churning releases more taste and flavor-producing nutrients from the food. In order to register the released nutrients with taste sensors, you have to bring the chewed portion of the food back on the tongue. Depending on the texture you may have to switch the rest of the food to the other side and repeat chewing and tasting until you have fully enjoyed each bite of food.
- If you swallow before enjoying your food, you're defeating the purpose of eating. You know from experience that you can enjoy food as paper thin as a slice of carrot, cucumber, or single potato chip in your mouth. In fact, if you put a stack of any of these in your mouth your taste buds will not come in contact with each individual slice.

Deciding What to Eat: The Subconscious Mind vs. the Conscious Mind

My other goal in this chapter is to help you become more conscious of your food choices. If you had to choose a pair of shoes, clothes, or other personal item from among 20 attractive and affordable possibilities, you would likely have some difficulty selecting a pair because all of the choices are appealing.

In contrast, if you had to choose food items from among 20 very enticing, affordable and attractive dishes, you would probably have less difficulty. This is because with items like clothes or shoes, your conscious mind makes a decision based on your color and style preferences and sense of comfort. However, when it comes to the food choice, your subconscious mind has the advantage of knowing both the current nutrient needs of your body and the approximate nutrient content of the foods presented. As soon as the food is shown, the subconscious mind evaluates every item in view. This evaluation is most effective if you have prior experience eating the foods because the subconscious is then capable of considering large numbers of nutrient combinations to satisfy the nutritional needs already known to the brain.

Armed with this information, your subconscious mind tries to influence your decision about what to eat. It has already determined which items contain the maximum number of relevant nutrients and relays the most promising ones to the conscious mind for selection. If multiple dishes are offered, the conscious mind has to decide which ones are most appealing and enjoyable to eat.

This coordination of the subconscious and conscious mind probably formed in humans to ensure our survival. We can imagine that without this screening by the subconscious mind, the conscious mind would have to spend a lot of time analyzing the importance of each item of food presented and its nutritional value to the body. The conscious mind could find valuable nutrients, some for immediate use and some for later use, in many of the items presented, but the time it takes to assess which foods are most valuable in the moment would take too long, just as it does when you are trying to choose a pair of shoes or a shirt from among too many choices. The analysis by the subconscious mind relieves the conscious mind of the need to evaluate each item of food based on beliefs and benefits.

The point of this is: When you find yourself intentionally thinking about a food or veering towards the choice of a restaurant or the selection of a specific food item, know that both your subconscious and conscious mind have guided you towards it. Use this information as a powerful clue to the fact that your brain is telling you that it needs certain nutritional elements found in that food item or type of cooking. Once you choose the dish you like, enjoy it to the fullest by eating slowly and consciously.

Conversely, when you find your conscious mind unable to make a choice about what to eat, it is often a sign that you do not need the nutrition at this time and, in fact, are not actually hungry. You may be acting out some other impulse that you have trained your subconscious mind to link to eating, such as eating as a reward for some activity, or eating from stress or worry.

Consuming Enough Micro vs. Macronutrients

Each food item you eat is a mixture of *macro-* and *micro*-nutrients existing in different combinations and ratios. Macronutrients are the larger, most common elements your body needs most. Micronutrients are those needed in small quantities but are nevertheless important in cell metabolism. The problem is, nutritional science does not yet have the tools to understand or study the long-term health impact of any food containing multiple nutrients. Projecting nutritional values of the foods that a given individual consumes is complicated by the specifics of the circumstances, such as the combination of foods eaten during a meal, since the metabolism of one nutritional element could impact the absorption of another.

Nevertheless, it is only logical that you should make an effort to eat a variety of foods to ensure you receive the greatest possible diversity of macro and micro nutrients possible. Our hunter-gatherer ancestors may have had to travel to many different areas to obtain food, especially micronutrients. They may have been compelled to eat more macronutrients such as carbohydrates, protein and fats to get enough of the needed micronutrients. In developed countries today where there is an abundant variety of foods in the local grocery store, micronutrient-rich foods are easily available, but this could change if the soil in which our food is grown is depleted of micronutrients, if the food comes from limited sources, or if processing depletes the food of micronutrients. These conditions could result in needing to eat an excess of macronutrients to get the needed micronutrients.

You don't need to understand the nutrient composition of any food you're eating if you let your subconscious mind and conscious sensory controls guide you to what items and how much to consume. Even if you're compelled to over-eat to meet the need for a particular micronutrient, your brain will help you terminate the meal when that need is met and compensate for the excess intake of other nutrients during subsequent meals. The most significant requirements are that you eat in response to hunger and that you consume a variety of natural, un-processed foods prepared simply and lovingly to preserve their nutrient values.

Give Eating Your Undivided Attention

Eating consciously is also about focusing your attention only on the meal. When people are unexpectedly interrupted, they not only perform less efficiently, but make more mistakes. An interruption forces the conscious part of the brain to shift attention to the new task. If you read a sentence in a book while listening to music, it's unlikely you'll grasp the meaning of the sentence.

Magnetic resonance imaging studies of brain activity show that when people concentrate simultaneously on two demanding tasks, total brain activity decreases rather than doubling. This could be because the conscious brain concentrates on one activity while delegating the second to the subconscious brain. While your brain is capable of multitasking, especially if you are familiar with the tasks, multitasking does not produce optimal performance. For example, when you pay attention to a conversation while eating, the latter is handed off to the subconscious part of your brain, which starts to process the signals coming from the taste and smell receptors in your mouth. Meanwhile, the conscious mind is distracted and cannot make the best choices about your food consumption.

When you eat with focus, your conscious mind sees any uneaten food on your plate, which the subconscious mind has already determined has nutritional value. However, the decision making part of your conscious mind can listen to signals coming from the brain and decide whether you are still in need of nutrients from that food. This area knows when the need for more of a nutrient is diminished due to adequate intake, and decreases the enjoyment.

However, if you are reading, watching TV, or performing an action while eating, your subconscious mind takes over and will keep eating because it knows the food has nutritional value and is simply following the past eating behavior already programmed in your brain. Your subconscious mind cannot pay attention to the signals from your mouth indicating a decreasing enjoyment of the food. If the subconscious mind is programmed to stop eating only when the plate is empty or your stomach signals indicate fullness, the result could be excess consumption relative to your immediate nutritional needs. In short, if you want to be confident in your ability to disregard food on your plate no matter how pleasing it looks or good it smells, you have to engage your conscious mind during the meal you're eating.

The evidence for this is solid. Increased food consumption while watching television has been identified as one of the key contributors to obesity. When you watch TV, your brain receives thousands of messages every second. Out of the multiple signals from the mouth, eyes and ears received by the brain during a meal while watching television, the brain is forced to select one to pay primary attention to, meanwhile scanning the rest of the information for other messages that could be valuable. As the images change on the TV, your brain is constantly shifting its orientation from the signals coming from the mouth to the rapidly changing sights and sounds on the screen. Out of all sensory input into your brain, you are programmed to receive messages most strongly through your eyes. If the mind pays no attention when you taste food, it is as if you have not tasted it and the quantity of food consumed is determined by your subconscious mind, as just explained. With repeated episodes of eating combined with attention-grabbing distractions, overeating becomes a behavior.

No matter how much you concentrate during your meal, other things such as reading, listening intensely to a conversation and watching an event make it difficult to regulate your intake based on sensory signals. The importance of this cannot be underestimated: Try to eat your meals in a calm, peaceful environment without distraction so that you can consciously focus on what you eat, how it tastes, and how much you are consuming.

The Importance of Noticing the Intensity of Your Enjoyment

If eating is about taking in nutrients for the survival of the body, stopping consumption should reflect when your body has received enough of the nutrients it needs. This takes time, however, given that an ordinary meal consists of multiple food groups, each containing a mixture of nutrients. This means that an accurate assessment of the composition and concentration of the nutrients consumed is not fully known to the brain until after the food is completely digested and absorbed, a process that can take hours. This is why the body supplies other signals that it is time to stop eating, as you learned earlier.

One of these signals is a change in the pleasantness of the food in your mouth. This is your clue to stop eating regardless of how much is left on the plate or the availability of more in the kitchen. In order to appreciate the drop in the intensity of pleasure related to the food you're eating, you first have to be aware of the pleasure of eating that food. This is how conscious eating helps you. Only when you pay attention to the food inside your mouth are you able to notice when its enjoyment is reduced. Multitasking and distractions during your meal keep your brain from noticing this transition. Although the concept of conscious eating and its variations may be familiar to you, what is different in this book is using the reduction in enjoyment of a meal as a means to regulate your food intake.

I cannot give you advice about how to rank your enjoyment of food in a way that can be measured. As yet, no system exists to help humans accurately quantify and express their enjoyment of eating in absolute numbers. The fact that almost every bite of food you eat has multiple nutrients, each stimulating the taste and smell receptors at different strengths, makes it even harder to notice when the intensity of your enjoyment changes. Perhaps the best scale you can use to assess the intensity of your enjoyment of eating is to compare each consecutive bite to the very first one you took. Unless you pay close attention, you will miss the diminishing intensity of enjoyment over the continuous stimulus of a meal, just as you would when listening to music and trying to read at the same time.

If you aren't sure whether you might be sensing lower enjoyment of your food, take a sip of water after each bite is chewed and swallowed to give your brain time to assess the situation, especially after eating complex carbohydrates. Warm water cleanses the taste buds better than cold water. When taste buds are already occupied with nutrients, they can't accept freshly released nutrients in the next bite of food. Washing the taste buds with water unclogs the taste pores to accept new molecules. If drinking so much is not amenable to you, just sip water every couple of minutes during the meal. The objective is not to fill your stomach with water but to cleanse your taste buds.

Note that drinking water does not remove the molecules that occupy the smell sensors in your nose. But if you breathe out through your nose, the air current will dislodge the nutrient molecules and carry them out. Another choice is to sip a warm drink such as hot tea, as the vapors from it can create the movement of warm air through the nose, facilitating the removal of molecules in the smell receptors.

Sipping wine also facilitates cleaning the smell receptors because of the alcohol vapors. It is not known, however, whether alcohol in the wine cleans the taste receptors as well. It's possible that those who savor wine and try to make distinctions between which grapes it was made from and its unique aromas and flavors pay more attention to the food they eat, although this has yet to be determined. By concentrating on changes in flavor due to the presence of alcohol, acid, fruitiness and tannin in each wine, wine connoisseurs become conscious of the minute differences in their food. If the wine is 'paired' with the food, meaning if it is chosen to compliment the flavors of the food, many people become even more aware of the harmonies among the tastes and smells in their mouth.

Developing your sense of taste to be more precise is possible because the processing structures in the neurons of your brain are capable of processing signals with very minimal difference. Most people can easily taste the difference between a peach and an apricot, a pear and an apple, and mahi-mahi and tilapia. But you can, with practice, equally train yourself to detect the minute differences between plums and pluots, Fuji and Gala apples, and brown and rainbow trout.

The brain also assigns different sets of neurons to process information based on priorities assigned to specific groups of signals. When you pay close attention to your food, the brain makes specific changes in the connecting pathways based on detailed differences in signals and priorities. In fact, it has been shown that when you pay attention to any task you're doing, the brain releases nerve growth agents that consolidate the connections between neurons, helping to wire them together for future coordinated action. In addition, nerve cells produce a number of proteins that allow information to be stored. This helps you remember the experience. This capability of the brain is very useful for establishing a new way of eating based on having an increasingly sophisticated palette.

What to Do about "Lingering Hunger"

As you transition into conscious and slow eating, you may feel that your hunger does not abate at the end of each meal even as you pay attention to the signals of satisfaction we've been discussing. One reason for this, confirmed by studies, is that during meals, most people can detect a reduction in the intensity of taste of a nutrient more than the intensity of their hunger. In other words, sometimes your hunger may not fully subside during a particular meal that you no longer enjoy the taste of. If you feel this, the solution is to tap into your will power for a few meals, because this sensation will subside as your brain learns that your hunger will be satisfied in the course of the next meals.

This brain training is similar to other repetitive activities in your life. Consider reading a very long book. You can read a little at a time, knowing that you can come back to it in the next sitting. Your brain does not experience any lack of enjoyment from reading in spurts. What you accomplish in subsequent readings is simply added onto the pages you read until you finish the book. Eating is the same. You may not consume all the nutrients you need during just one meal, but there will be other meals to come. Once your brain can be assured of the fact that you'll have opportunities to eat again, you'll be able to stop eating before you feel full. Slowly, this new way of eating will become natural.

In many ways, this is not so different from what you may already do. When you eat a small breakfast, you may already tell yourself that it is enough as lunch will soon follow. Similarly, if you eat a large breakfast, you are okay with just a small lunch, knowing that dinner will fill in your hunger gap. In short, the nutrition monitoring system detects not only what the body absorbed during a meal but also what was not acquired. If you can begin to apply this same thinking to all your meals, you will soon train yourself to be satisfied with a smaller volume of food at each meal, knowing you will consume more nutrition at a later meal.

Gaining Confidence in Your New Eating Behavior

Each time you eat, you have the opportunity to embed the new way of eating in your brain. The key to establishing a new eating behavior is to change each and every element that defines your past processes of eating. You can force your brain to concentrate on your new behavior by replacing as many of the practices that remind you of your old eating pattern with new ones.

For example, drink water instead of your favorite drink. If you are already drinking water with your meal, try a different type, like filtered, carbonated or bottled, or drink warm water rather than cold. Use a new glass for your water. If you have a favorite chair or place you sit to eat your meal, change it. Try new recipes instead of making the same ones over and over. Use new utensils and a new plate. Buy smaller portions of meat and fish. Take smaller bites than you did before. Chew each bite more times than before.

In order to get back to and maintain your authentic weight, you need to create new habits that reinforce your goal to regulate your food intake. Here is a summary checklist of the many things you learned so far in this chapter:

- Activate the sensory mechanisms in your body that allow you to enjoy your food and pay attention to the signals of hunger and satisfaction. Following these will allow you to consume food with only occasional intake in excess of your immediate nutritional needs.
- Let your subconscious mind help you to select food based on your internal need for specific nutrients and the potential availability of the nutrients in the items presented.
- Limit your selection of food items to those that require chewing before swallowing. This will help ensure that the nutritional molecules of food register in your mouth and contribute to your enjoyment of the food.
- As much as possible, serve yourself the type and quantity of each item of food you want to eat rather than letting someone else serve you. This is to prevent the temptation of eating all that's served in order to avoid wasting food or to please the host.
- Chew each bite of food thoroughly to release and enjoy the nutrients.

- Consume all liquids except water by sipping. This will ensure more registration of dissolved nutrients.
- Always leave a portion of food on your plate as a token of your accomplishment.
- When you eat out, try a new restaurant or order a new entrée.
- Any time you think of food, think of eating it slowly. Form a mental picture of each chewing motion and of enjoying the taste. Each time you do this your brain connections change. If you can learn to imagine terminating a meal based on taste satisfaction, you can more easily actually do it during a meal.
- When you travel or go on a vacation, you probably look forward to enjoying as much of your experience as possible. However, you have to bring the same mindset to each meal when you travel.

Make these changes one at a time. With each change you will begin to establish new neural connections and create a pathway that makes your new eating behavior the automatic response. Each time you repeat the new way of eating, these connections are strengthened.

It can take weeks before you learn the new eating habit. It can take months of concentration and practice before the habit becomes automatic. However, as you become a veteran at it, you will learn how to listen closely to your brain and recognize what it tells you. This is possible because you have reset the goal of eating to meet the nutrient needs of your body, not to fill your belly. Your brain will direct what conscious and unconscious actions are needed to accomplish that objective during each meal. As you get good at this skill, you will gain more self-control to put down the fork and end your meal any time you want.

Consciously exerting this control is what you need to do to maintain your authentic weight. In order to be successful in this objective, you must work out a plan to be aware of not only every bite of food, but also of each chewing motion. You will most likely need to exercise self-discipline to carry out this plan so you can experience several meals in full while practicing it. It won't help if you quit before you start getting results.

Remember that all these years, you practiced a certain way of consuming all the nutrients your body needed. It's only natural for your brain to resist learning other ways of accomplishing the same objective. This makes it harder for the new ways to compete with something at which you're already proficient. During the early stages of practicing this method, you'll catch yourself falling back to the old way of eating. This is because most of the pathways that were used for the old eating habit are still in the brain, available for the subconscious mind.

Also, one of the major reasons for sliding back to your old way of eating is consumption of foods that requires practically no chewing. The surest way to get back on track is deliberately selecting only foods with texture, paying attention to each chewing motion and enjoying the nutrients released in the mouth.

Use these moments of recognition as opportunities to remind yourself that your old way of eating was based on the belief that the more you ate, the more you enjoyed your food. This notion may have started in your infancy when your mother coaxed you to take one more bite to finish what was on the plate. A babysitter or day care worker may have reinforced this by telling your mother how good you were on that day because you ate well, and that message made your mother happy. A relationship between the quantity of food eaten, being a good person, and producing happiness could have been established from that time onwards.

Each time you catch yourself going back to the old way of eating, use the opportunity to feel satisfied that you were able at least to identify and correct that old eating habit. In order to establish the new way of eating, you have to replace most of the signals produced in your mouth by the old way of eating with new ones. Otherwise, the brain can easily go back to the old way of eating as soon as it detects familiar signals coming from the mouth. For example, if many food items are familiar to you, it's easy for the old way of eating to emerge without your awareness, unless you change to new food items just to help establish a new way of eating.

The most important time during the transition learning period is most likely your evening meal, since the largest meal of the day for most people in the US is dinner. This means you need to be especially vigilant during this meal to eat slowly and consciously, savoring your food. Pay attention to the size of the bite, be aware of the feel of the food in the mouth, and enjoy the flavors and the warmth or coldness of the food. Check your speed of chewing and the movement of the food inside your mouth and pay attention to when you stop chewing, or swallow the chewed portion. If you do these actions wrong, you can trigger your old way of eating.

Although smaller bite size and slower chewing speed are powerful reminders that you are undertaking a new way of eating, the most critical factor in firmly establishing the habit is the feeling of satisfaction you generate each time you do it right. Repeated feelings of satisfaction will establish in your memory bank that your new way of eating will help you preserve harmony among all the organs in your body. After practicing the new way of eating for a while, you'll be able to catch yourself before you even start going down the wrong path. Once the new way of eating is fully established, you'll only need to correct your way of eating occasionally because most of the time you'll be eating the right way.

As you become efficient in executing this plan, you will feel hungry at different times than in the past. Sometimes you'll feel hungry earlier, especially if you have been physically active. Sometimes the reverse will happen. This change in your hunger is proof that your internal regulatory system is sensitive to the reduced level of stored nutrients, since you are eating less and perhaps losing weight. But keep in mind that your new eating behavior is more efficient, treating your body like a well-run factory. By arranging for parts to be shipped to the assembly plant on a timely basis, only as need arises, the company can operate with less stored parts and less need for a storage area.

Don't Rely on Third Party Programs and Prepackaged Foods

I hope this chapter has shown you that changing your eating behavior must involve consciously making an effort to alter the neural pathways in your brain. You need to establish and reinforce new connections in the brain that support the elements of conscious eating—chewing slowly, tasting your food, paying attention to the signals from your mouth, and so on. The best way to achieve and maintain your authentic weight and cut out excess food consumption is to relearn this new eating behavior to replace your old one.

You might be tempted to use prepackaged foods or to follow instructions from one of the corporate weight loss management program to help you accomplish your goals. However, I would strongly discourage you from doing this.

When you give the responsibility of determining what you eat and how much you eat to someone else, someone who has no intimate knowledge of your bodily needs, you lose the opportunity to retrain your brain. This is why nearly all of these programs fail in the long run. People who rely on outside instructions and prepackaged foods are unable to form new neural pathways that create a new eating behavior using real food. The moment they stop using prepackaged foods and go back to eating on their own, they revert to old eating patterns—not chewing their food, not tasting the nutrients, not letting the signals from their mouth and nose reach the brain to help them notice the moment of satisfaction.

My recommendation is that you take responsibility for changing your own eating behavior. It is far better to prepare and eat your own food, using your own recipes, so you can learn to eat right no matter what you consume. Doing it yourself makes you far more conscious of what foods and how much of them you eat rather than sitting down to a plastic tray of food you have selected just because it contains less than 300 calories or less than 5 grams of fat. Developing the skills and ability to control your own eating can be met more easily by letting your internal regulatory system be in charge rather than some external system of food management or supplements.

I suggest you not depend on labels indicating energy content, fat grams, percentage of added sugar, serving size, average recommended amount, etc. Your conscious mind can learn to concentrate on enjoying every morsel of food that you consume to meet the objective of adjusting the meal size. When you let another person or organization prescribe what you eat, you undermine your ability to make your own food selections. Your mealtime is your own to enjoy. Do not allow anyone to take that away from you.

Healthy Living, Diabetes Free

Whatever your current age, the recommendations in this book will help you age more happily. When you achieve your goal to rediscover and maintain your authentic weight, you will find yourself having more energy, feeling better about yourself, and finally enjoying one of the most meaningful activities of life—eating. Each meal will become a sensory experience that delights you and reinforces your ability to eat for nourishment and avoid excess food intake.

My interest in this area was prompted by my curiosity as to why most toddlers and young children can eat and not gain weight or become prediabetic. I found out they are naturally inclined to follow the signals from their body telling them when they are hungry, when they need certain nutrients, and when they are satisfied. This is the evolutionary human approach to eating right.

I am suggesting that you return to this "toddler" way of eating. As a toddler you knew that at mealtimes you experienced the pleasure of eating. A toddler eats based on the feeling of hunger sensation and can't be hurried, even when encouraged to speed up the process. How much you ate as a toddler was based on your own satisfaction in spite of enticements and threats from caregivers.

The most significant challenge for you as an adult is to achieve the same mental framework of relaxed enjoyment during mealtimes. Of course, as an adult, you may often be constrained by obligations and pressures that prevent you from eating like a toddler. You have probably become conditioned to eat a certain volume of food based on the time of day and location of the meal, such as a cafeteria, restaurant, or home, or the occasion, such as sporting events, movies, formal celebrations or outdoor gatherings.

However, you can retrain your brain and become conscious of your eating behavior. Knowing the natural mechanism that underlies the hunger instinct should give you the confidence to apply these principles. You will need this understanding to overcome challenges, mostly external, and to learn the skills to prevent the development of Type 2 diabetes. You can develop the smarts to become immune to food and image marketing and cultivate a lifestyle in which you eat what you enjoy, enjoy what you eat, and eat less of what you can't enjoy.

As you get in touch with your authentic weight and practice conscious eating at every meal, you will find yourself automatically eating right and enjoying it more. You will chew your food with appreciation for its nutrients. You will taste more of the flavors, spices, textures, and unique qualities in each recipe. You will be paying attention to what your brain tells you about your hunger and satisfaction. You will become more conscious of what to eat and how much of it, and will reconnect with your body's natural rhythms for eating and activity.

Being in touch with your body is one of the keys to healthy aging. The more aware you are of your authentic weight and nutritional needs, the better you will be at self-regulating your health as you age. For instance, as your energy expenditure changes over time, you will be better at sensing when your need for energy nutrients should be increased or reduced. You may grow old, but you will not grow fat or obese. You may slow down, but you will know how to feed your internal organs properly with the variety of nutrients they need to stay healthy and functioning. When you become deeply in touch with your body in the present moment, all your meals will become more satisfying and enjoyable. Living in the present is the toddler way, but it is also the natural way to prevent diabetes.

KEY POINTS

- Your mission during a meal should be to eat what you enjoy and, more importantly, to enjoy what you eat. Return to the "toddler" way of eating, when you knew the pleasure of eating and ate enough to supply your body with nutrients without overeating.

- The best way to retrain yourself in a new way of eating is to start with the act of chewing. Take small bites, put food on your tongue, and enjoy the food in your mouth. Chew with the conscious intention of experiencing the nutrients in food on your taste and smell receptors. Eating slowly and consciously are perhaps the ultimate keys to health. Your ability to assess the nutrients in your food is directly proportional to the amount of time nutrients remain in contact with your taste and smell receptors.

- Don't give away the responsibility of determining what you eat and how much you eat to someone else through corporate diet programs, diet mixes, and prepackaged foods.

- If you lose weight and see a lowering of your blood sugar (confirmed with A1C blood tests), maintain your commitment to your new eating habits. Don't be fooled into complacency, thinking you can go back to eating grain-based carbohydrates and overconsuming at meals. Respect your body and its warning message that if you go back to your old habits, you will revert back to being prediabetic or diabetic.

EAT AND ENJOY TO CONTROL YOUR BLOOD SUGAR

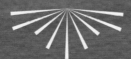

HOW YOU EAT MATTERS MORE THAN WHAT YOU EAT

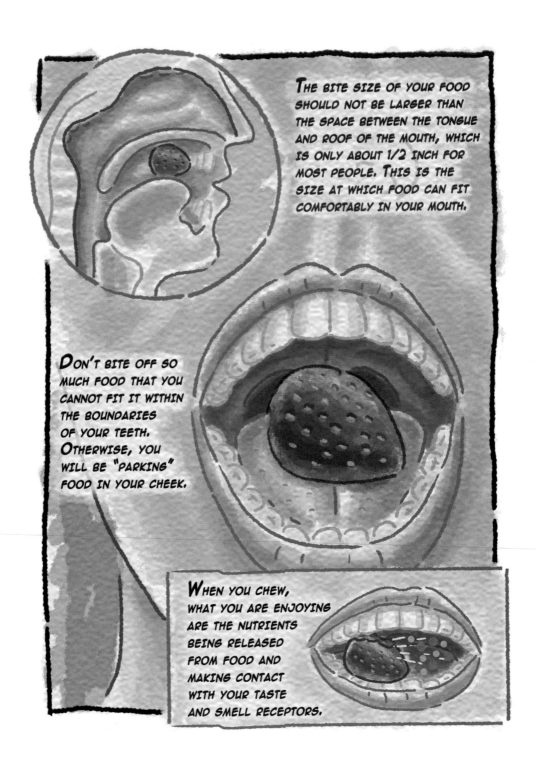

THE BITE SIZE OF YOUR FOOD SHOULD NOT BE LARGER THAN THE SPACE BETWEEN THE TONGUE AND ROOF OF THE MOUTH, WHICH IS ONLY ABOUT 1/2 INCH FOR MOST PEOPLE. THIS IS THE SIZE AT WHICH FOOD CAN FIT COMFORTABLY IN YOUR MOUTH.

DON'T BITE OFF SO MUCH FOOD THAT YOU CANNOT FIT IT WITHIN THE BOUNDARIES OF YOUR TEETH. OTHERWISE, YOU WILL BE "PARKING" FOOD IN YOUR CHEEK.

WHEN YOU CHEW, WHAT YOU ARE ENJOYING ARE THE NUTRIENTS BEING RELEASED FROM FOOD AND MAKING CONTACT WITH YOUR TASTE AND SMELL RECEPTORS.

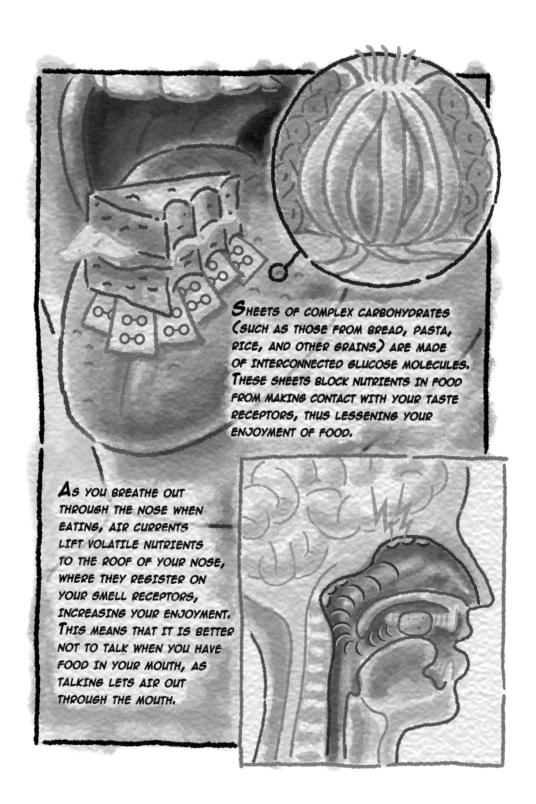

Sheets of complex carbohydrates (such as those from bread, pasta, rice, and other grains) are made of interconnected glucose molecules. These sheets block nutrients in food from making contact with your taste receptors, thus lessening your enjoyment of food.

As you breathe out through the nose when eating, air currents lift volatile nutrients to the roof of your nose, where they register on your smell receptors, increasing your enjoyment. This means that it is better not to talk when you have food in your mouth, as talking lets air out through the mouth.

Principles of Eat, Chew, Live

- Chew slowly. Enjoy your food before swallowing it.

- Eating less of what you can't enjoy reduces weight and prevents diabetes.

- It is more natural to get your vitamins from vegetables than from fortified grain products.

- It is more enjoyable to get your carbohydrate from fruits than from grain products.

- You are more likely to develop diabetes because of the fat created from carbohydrate than from fat you enjoy in its natural form.

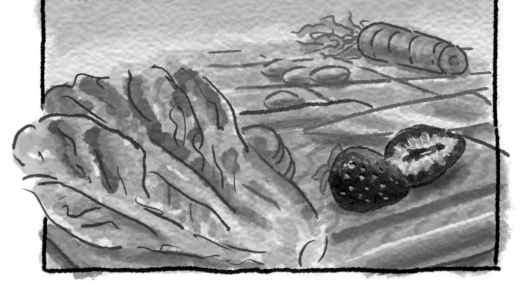

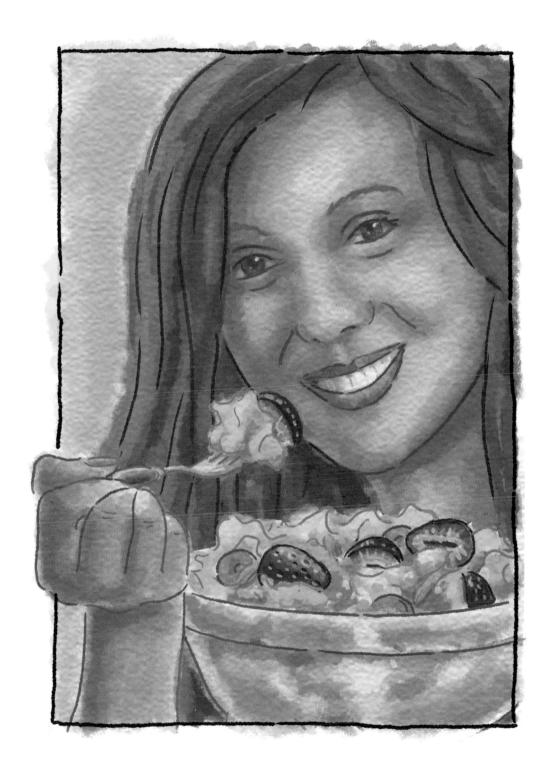

SEE HOW YOU EAT

Take a video of yourself eating. Analyze whether you are:

- taking large bites of food or small ones?

- not chewing enough before you swallow?

- talking with food in your mouth? or

- not drinking water often enough?

Then watch your video and see if you can determine some changes that will help you to eat more consciously and enjoy more of what you eat.

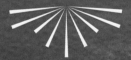

CHAPTER 31

Adjusting Your Diabetic Medications

Your body treats the nutrients glucose and cholesterol in a similar fashion, as explained in Chapter 7. However, the irony is that it is simpler and more straightforward to control high blood glucose levels, reverse prediabetes and prevent diabetes than it is to control high cholesterol levels.

Almost all the glucose in your blood comes from the food you eat, especially grain-based carbohydrate. Although your liver also makes glucose from amino acids not used for protein production, it is largely overconsumption of carbohydrate that drives high blood sugar. In contrast, cholesterol in your blood comes not only from what you eat but also from what your liver manufactures under the direction of the genes you inherited. (Proof of this is the fact that strict vegetarians who don't eat meat still produce cholesterol in the liver.)

Endocrinologists, by setting the criteria for the diagnosis and management, have made medical treatment of Type 2 diabetes more complicated than it ought to be. For example, if your blood sugar levels keep climbing in spite of taking medications, you may be told, without any additional testing, that it is not an indication of your diabetes getting worse. It is because, they tell you, your medications "stopped working" for reasons diabetes experts don't fully understand. If you ask whether you should reduce the amount of carbohydrate in your diet, you will be reassured that carbohydrate is an important nutrient and, as long as the amount per meal/snack does not exceed the recommended amount, you don't need to reduce it. Instead, diabetes experts may insist that you need to change your medication, use a different combination of medications, or begin taking insulin, along with more frequent tests at home and in the laboratory to monitor blood sugar levels.

None of those three solutions is accurate. If your goal is to lower your blood sugar, reduce or get off of your blood sugar medications, and even reverse a diagnosed case of diabetes, you should consider the following steps:

1. Eliminate grain products from your daily diet. Stop eating bread, pastas, rice, pastries and cakes, and other elements of meals made with starch. **Making lentils the source of carbohydrate for your body is the most effective treatment to reduce elevated blood sugar if you have prediabetes or diabetes.** Legumes such as lentils were part of the human diet long before agriculture became established as an integral part of human life. The variety of lentils available in different parts of the world provides a wider source of needed nutrients compared to the smaller number of cultivated grains. Remember that, during infancy, most of the excess glucose that was converted to fat in your body came from milk. Your body was able to make use of the stored fat for your growth, mostly vertical as you gain height. During adult life, excess glucose, mostly from grains, accumulates in the body as fat and is responsible for your horizontal growth as you gain weight. Since the accumulation of fat leads to the subsequent elevation of blood glucose in a manner that is directly proportional to your intake of carbohydrate, you will see an almost immediate reduction in your blood sugar level once you eliminate grain products.

2. Check your fasting blood sugar daily at home until the levels stabilize within the normal range.

3. Let your doctor know that you have changed your diet. Discuss the recommendations in this book with your physician and seek his or her help to lower the dosage of your diabetic medications.

4. Have your doctor check your fasting blood sugar and triglyceride levels through a blood lab. You may have to pay for this as your insurance carrier may not approve payment if you are tested more often than they allow. Consult your doctor to decide on the frequency of this test.
5. Your doctor may want to continue testing your A1C levels every 3 months until he or she is satisfied that you are no longer a diabetic.

How fast your blood sugar will drop is unpredictable because it depends on many factors, including the amount of carbohydrate you are consuming not just in grains, but in vegetables, fruits, dairy products, and natural sugars. It also depends on how much glucose is already attached to various body proteins. Just as glucose attaches to the red blood cell protein (A1C), it can also attach to other proteins in the body. These will become detached, reenter the bloodstream and elevate your blood sugar level temporarily until they are burned away. Fortunately, as your fat cells empty out from your lower consumption of carbohydrate, they will begin to accommodate more triglycerides. This means less fatty acids will be available for muscles to use as fuel and so they will begin burning the glucose in your blood instead, lowering your blood sugar. Yet another possibility is that you may experience lowering of your blood sugar without significant weight loss because you did not have a lot of glucose attached to other proteins in the body.

However, keep in mind also that your liver can produce glucose from amino acids. Therefore, if you consume proteins in excess of what your body can use, it can result in elevating glucose in the blood. A lower carbohydrate intake doesn't mean you can overeat protein-rich foods such as meat, as some diets have recommended. This is especially true if you eat a high-protein meal in the evening because it is natural for your body to release growth hormone and cortisol in the early morning hours. This can prompt the liver to convert the amino acids from your meal into glucose and cause elevated blood sugar in the morning. In addition, your body can also absorb glucose that you digested from the glycogen stored in the meat you consumed. For example, when blubber, the traditional diet of the Inuit was analyzed, it was found to contain as much as 8 to 30 percent glycogen. So remember what counts is changing your approach to eating and learning not to overconsume.

Getting off of diabetes medication is also a function of how fast your pancreas adjusts the amount of insulin released to reflect your lower total intake of carbohydrate during each meal. In the beginning of the process, the pancreas may continue to release the same amount of insulin as before because of its previous programming. This can result in a lower than expected blood sugar level until the pancreas is reset. Provided your pancreas is still capable of releasing adequate amounts of insulin and has not been exhausted from past prolonged use of medications that overstimulated its insulin-producing cells, a reset will occur. The irony is that individuals who were put on insulin injections may have an advantage over those who took oral medications because their insulin-producing cells were spared from overstimulation and possible exhaustion.

Be aware though that if you are already on insulin injections, stopping the intake of grain and grain products may necessitate a lowering of the insulin dosage to prevent hypoglycemia from happening at the time of peak insulin action. In addition, significant absorption of alcohol or sedatives coinciding with the peak action of insulin in the body may put your life in danger by interfering with the awareness of the symptoms of hypoglycemia. If you routinely take insulin before a meal to control the post-meal elevation of blood glucose, you may want to wait and check your sugar level two hours after eating before deciding the dosage. Keep in mind that a blood sugar level up to 140md/dl is considered normal.

As you contemplate getting off your medications for diabetes, it is motivating to imagine all the benefits. First, changing your diet to lower your blood sugar can have an additional pay-off: you may be able to stop taking medication for high blood pressure. This is because the elevation of blood glucose is also closely associated with an elevation of sodium ions in your body. Both of these nutrients require water to stay in solution. Because of this, people with high blood sugar have a higher blood volume, which leads to developing or worsening high blood pressure. Lowering your blood sugar can therefore reduce your blood pressure.

Second, committing to a new diet will give you the additional benefit of a lower blood triglyceride count. Recall that triglyceride produced in the liver from excess glucose can either stay in the blood or be stored, leading to weight gain and/or central obesity, based on the location of storage. This means that eliminating grain products from your diet could help you not only to reduce medications you are taking to lower your blood sugar, but also those to control many other associated health conditions.

Next, you will not have to spend money on medications. In addition, because the most common forms of hypoglycemia in Type 2 diabetes occur as a complication of treatments with insulin or oral medications, you will experience fewer hypoglycemic episodes as you reduce your blood sugar medications.

Finally, consider the joy of the weight loss you will naturally experience by altering your consumption habits and cutting out carbohydrate. You will be able to live free of the fear of spending the rest of your life coping with diabetes. And most of all, consider the freedom you will experience in choosing when and what you want to eat. Think how much you will enjoy eating without the restraints imposed by medications, approved foods, or prescribed meal schedules.

KEY POINTS

- Making changes in two patterns of behavior—limiting your consumption of grain products and eating consciously—can help you to lower your diabetes medications.

- Selecting lentils as your source of carbohydrate is the most effective treatment to reduce blood sugar if you have prediabetes or diabetes.

- If an experience such as a stressful event or illness sidetracks your attempt to change your eating behavior, restart one simple step by one simple step, each giving you more and more confidence to return to your commitment.

As a high school and college athlete my greatest challenge was trying to gain weight beyond my 175 pounds, but by age 58, I weighed 234. I realized that I was likely headed towards Type 2 diabetes. This book has been a real catalyst to change. I understand now that I don't need to eat much to meet my body's real requirements. To my amazement, the hunger waves that once hit me subsided and I started losing weight. I don't feel deprived. I look better and I have significantly more energy. I have a growing sense of confidence that I can have a long life of good health without the curse of Type 2 diabetes.

Eric, Overweight Adult, Oregon

CHAPTER 32

Frequently Asked Questions about Type 2 Diabetes, Weight and Eating

1. How can I work with my doctor if I begin implementing the ideas in this book to reverse my high blood sugar or Type 2 diabetes?

Every person is different and, since I'm not your physician, I can only provide general advice. That said, I recommend that you discuss your desire to reverse your diabetes with your doctor. You must take responsibility for the changes you make in your diet and in your medications, preferably in consultation with your doctor. I'd suggest letting him or her know that you have read this book and that it presents a new theory on the cause of Type 2 diabetes that counters the accepted theory of insulin resistance.

Whether or not your doctor is willing to help you, you can still begin implementing the recommendations I make in Part 3 to reconnect with your authentic weight, and in Part 4 to overhaul your eating habits. This advice will help you no matter what your circumstances are. Avoid grain-based products and consume a variety of fresh fruits and vegetables to obtain your nutrients. Reflect on the reasons and circumstances in which you tend to overeat—and begin paying attention to your hunger and satisfaction signals so you can eat for nutrition, not to fill your stomach. Seek to empty your fat cells and lose weight if you need to, but be patient with yourself. One pound a week of weight loss is fine. Follow the recommendations I make about eating slowly and consciously. Chew your food to savor it and give your brain a chance to register the nutrients in your mouth. Relearn to eat as you did when you were a child, eating only when hungry and only enough to be satisfied. Look forward to each meal and enjoy your food.

Work with your doctor to obtain regular A1C blood tests every 3 months to check if your blood sugar is becoming lower. Also ask your doctor to test your triglyceride levels, since these are an indication of the amount of fatty acids in your blood. Keep in mind that your diet of fruits, vegetables, dairy, and natural sugars will impact how fast your blood sugar drops. If you are making progress in lowering your blood sugar and triglycerides, create a plan with your doctor to adjust your medications as suggested in Chapter 31. Be sure to reread pages 267-268 for some important information about how to lower your medication dosage, in conjunction with your doctor's recommendations.

Be aware that it will take time for most doctors to adjust to the concept that diabetes can be controlled and even reversed with the lifestyle changes described in this book.

2. If my blood sugar goes down in my next A1C test, can I go back to eating grain-based products such as bread, rice, and corn?

The answer is no. Lowering your blood sugar, even if your doctor agrees that you are no longer prediabetic or diabetic, does not mean you can revert to your old eating habits. It was those habits of overconsumption, especially of grain-based foods, that led to high blood sugar. It would be a mistake to think that now that your fat cells must be empty, you can fill them again. Your commitment to being diabetes-free is a lifelong commitment to respect your body and eat slowly and consciously, putting nutrition ahead of filling your stomach with carbs so you can feel full.

3. My father and mother are overweight, but my brother is not. I feel that I have inherited the obesity genes as I'm having a hard time losing pounds and finding my authentic weight. What should I do?

As much as 70 percent of the differences in weight between individuals may be accounted for by genetic factors. However, genes are not solely responsible for the trend we see among millions of people who are gaining weight and becoming obese. Our genes have not changed substantially during the past 50 years, but the prevalence of obesity and persons who are overweight has risen significantly over the same period. We must be honest about this: it is largely due to overconsumption of high carb foods and sugars that fill people's fat cells and creates the stage for the global obesity trend.

Given this, your parents may be overweight because of their diet and overconsumption. You may have learned your eating habits from them. Reflect on your family's food choices and meals when you were growing up. Evaluate whether your current eating habits reflect what and how much you learned to eat at meals. When you are stressed, are you turning to "comfort" foods that you grew up with? Begin modifying your eating habits by following Parts 3 and 4 of this book. See if cutting out grain-based products, sugars and salt help you lose weight. Try this approach for 3 to 6 months, and you may discover that your genetic ancestry is not entirely responsible for your weight or your ability to lose pounds.

The increasing scientific discoveries in genetics will help people gain a better understanding of the role of their genes in their health. Genetic information can reveal your capacity to store excess nutrients and your potential for developing complications associated with weight gain, such as high cholesterol or diabetes. Genetic information will someday allow doctors to identify the most effective therapy each person needs based on inherited mechanisms of disease treatment. However, a better understanding of genetic information will not alter the basic preventive strategy for diabetes: food intake must match nutrient utilization, otherwise you will once again fill your fat cells, gain weight, and create the conditions for the fatty acid burn switch, leaving glucose in your blood. In other words, although genes determine your potential, they do not control your destiny. Just as you can decide the speed with which you drive a car, you can control how fast you fill up your potential fat storage capacity.

4. Humans have been eating grains for millennia. Today many nutritional experts say that eating "whole grains" are beneficial

because of the vitamins they offer. Why do you recommend not eating grain-based foods?

It is true that humans have eaten grains for thousands of years. The main reason why grains should no longer play a key role in diets today is because grains have become the leading cause of high blood sugar and diabetes. In Chapter 22, I discuss how modern milling techniques have made flour-based products ubiquitous. In the U.S. and in many other cultures, food intake of adults now includes up to 50 percent of daily calories from grain-based products. Breads, pasta, noodles, rice, dry cereals, cookies, cakes, doughnuts, and many other grain-containing products are consumed daily. Wheat flour is also used as filler or thickener in sauces and gravies. In short, humans are consuming far more complex carbohydrates from grains than in the past. This is why the incidence of Type 2 diabetes, as mentioned in Chapter 22, increased over 160 percent in the US from 1980 to 2012. It is also why diabetes is on the rise in countries like India and China that are increasingly marketing mass-produced and heavily marketed grains and grain-based breads, sweets, and packaged foods to their populations. In addition, in Chapter 24, I explain how the consumption of grain-based carbohydrate starting in infancy leads to a lifelong preference for salty foods, which in turn leads to craving more foods made with carbohydrates.

Human lifespans are also longer, providing decades more time to fill up fat cells and create the conditions for the "fatty acid burn switch." This may be why 1 in 4 adults over age 65 in the US has diabetes.

Despite this, the food industry and government-supported agricultural subsidies for grain farmers continue to market grains. However, it is just advertising, not science, to claim that "whole grain," "multigrain," "no cholesterol," "gluten free," "fortified with vitamins and minerals" and "no high-fructose corn syrup" makes products better for you. If they contain any type of grain (wheat, oats, barley, rye, and other cereal crops, as well as rice and corn), they are still foods that will elevate your blood sugar.

If you accept my theory that the cause of Type 2 diabetes is filling one's fat cells, causing your muscle cells to begin burning fatty acids rather than glucose, then there can only be one conclusion: you must reduce, if not eliminate, grain-based carbohydrates from your diet. This stops diabetes from starting, which is much better for your health than taking medications to reduce already high blood sugar.

5. Are you really expecting me to forego eating cereal for breakfast, an occasional sandwich for lunch, and foods like pasta, pita bread, tortilla, and rolls for dinner?

This question is just another way of rephrasing the previous question—and the answer is still yes. Avoiding grain-based carbs is the best way to empty your fat cells. By doing so, the glucose your body does not immediately use after a meal, which is converted to triglycerides, has somewhere to be stored. You can also empty your fat cells by exercising, but as I wrote in Chapter 18, most older adults cannot burn more calories by exercising than they consume in a day.

To stick with this change in diet, you will need to listen to another part of your brain that recognizes the long-term dangers of having diabetes for the rest of your life. You will need to break decades-old patterns of stimulus-response, such as reaching for coffee and a sweet roll, bagel, bread and jam first thing in the morning when you're hungry. You will need to regain control of your food choices and create new patterns of behavior, using the ways I recommend in Chapter 29. It's fine to consume a small quantity of grain-based products, even on a daily basis, or a larger quantity occasionally when you don't have a choice. Keep in mind that the frequency and quantity of grain-based foods consumed over a period of time is what fills up your fat storage capacity.

As humans, we are capable of change. We can unlearn patterns of thinking. We can replace old work and play habits with new ones, and continuously change interactions with people close to us. Think of changing your breakfast food choices as just taking a different road to work. See lunch as a chance to try new types of freshly prepared vegetables and fruits. Shop for dinner with an eye to trying out new recipes and using new spices to flavor your meal and savoring the different taste and smell sensations. You may find that giving up rice, corn, and grain-based breads and other preparations is far easier than you thought. More importantly, you will not feel hungry any earlier than before, even though you did not fill up your stomach during a meal, and your energy level will be the same as it was after eating the way you used to.

6. There are many types of prepackaged low-carb food products available. What is wrong with eating those?

I am against relying on prepackaged products to learn how to eat well to prevent high blood sugar and diabetes. Not only do these products possibly contain other ingredients that your body may not need, such as fillers and artificial ingredients, but they seldom have the same nutritional value as freshly prepared foods. In addition, most prepackaged foods are high in salt that your body may have trouble getting rid of.

As one of the four key points in this book has suggested, your brain monitors your body's nutrient needs. The micro- and macronutrients found in fresh fruits, vegetables, meats and dairy products are those that the brain seeks to identify and send to your body's cells as needed. Prepackaged foods may supply some of these nutrients, but in many instances, the cooking and/or freezing preparation of these products alters their nutrient composition.

I am convinced that you will enjoy your meals and be more successful at changing your eating habits for life if you emphasize freshly prepared foods that have been made with fresh seasonal ingredients.

7. Are fatty foods like meat and dairy products better to eat than carbohydrate-containing foods made from grains?

As I discuss in Chapter 21, beginning in the 1950s, researchers began citing fats as the cause of heart disease and atherosclerosis. Fat appeared to be leading contributor to health problems in the US, and a health campaign encouraged Americans to eat less fat and more carbohydrates. A healthy breakfast was considered to be cereals, muffins, or oatmeal; a healthy lunch, whole grain bread with lean meat; and dinner recommendations were small portions of meat with a larger serving of potatoes, rice, or corn, plus a vegetable. However, current research suggests that fats have taken more blame as a contributor to disease than they deserve. This is not to suggest that anyone revert to consuming large amounts of fats.

The body needs fats such as cholesterol. In general, 25 percent of the cholesterol in your body comes from dietary cholesterol. The liver produces the rest from fatty acids. The body also needs fat-associated nutrients. People enjoy eating foods with fat, oil and butter, despite the fact that without salt or spices, fats don't taste pleasant. The variety and flexibility of oil and fat and their ability to attach to different flavor-stimulating chemicals make them a favorite tool of all cooks.

My position is that an excess of carbohydrates in one's diet, especially from grain-based products, provides a greater risk than fat in its natural form, as it increasingly leads to high blood triglycerides, fatty acids, sugar and diabetes. For example, more than 50 percent of the energy in an average adult diet today comes from grain-based carbohydrates. I am in favor of a diet that contains an extensive variety of fresh foods, including vegetables, fruits, meat, fish, nuts, and dairy. If a person chooses to be vegan, then the diet must include sources of protein, vitamins, minerals, and other nutrients that are not obtained from meats and dairy.

Finally, based on the concept of eating for nutrients that this book presents, I remind you that it is not a particular food group that is important in creating satisfaction during a meal, but the registration of a sufficient amount of needed nutrients with taste and smell receptors.

8. It has been stated that the body is already dehydrated by the time the sensation of thirst is felt. Should I try to prevent dehydration by drinking even before I feel thirsty?

The body regulates the entry of water in cells based on its utilization. If cells can use water, it is allowed to enter, but otherwise it's not. It's true that when the thirst sensation is generated, there is a reduction of eight percent in the fluid volume in the body. This is because of the way the body's control mechanisms work. The deficit creates signals to the brain from receptors in charge of monitoring a molecule needed in the body. The brain in turn generates a response to correct the deficit. This is as true for water as it for breathing to acquire more oxygen and eating to get needed nutrients.

Although the body could be deficient in water by the time you feel thirsty, your water need depends on the amount of water you lose daily through urination, perspiration, and water evaporation through breathing. All these variables can be influenced by environmental temperature, physical activity, and the type of food you consume. In other words, it is difficult to predetermine the exact quantity of water a person may need on any given day. The consumption of caffeine or other diuretics will accelerate water loss. If you don't drink enough to replace what you lose, your body pulls water from the cells, causing dryness and interfering with natural functions to a degree that depends on how deficient in water you are. Your brain is aware of the degree of hydration in the body and produces the sensation of thirst in time to prevent the possibility of dehydration. As long as you drink enough water to quench your thirst, you're likely meeting your water needs

9. As I get older, can changes in my metabolism make it difficult for me to maintain my authentic weight?

The term metabolism may be understood in two different ways. The first refers to metabolism as the amount of work that can be done with a certain amount of food. In this sense, during your lifetime, the amount of work your body gets out of each ounce of food, the efficiency of energy extraction, does not significantly change as you age. Each person is different, however. An automobile with a gas tank capacity of 10 gallons and an engine giving 25 miles per gallon of gas can travel 250 miles on a full tank. However, a car whose engine gets 30 miles per gallon will be able to travel 300 miles. (The analogy to humans would work better if any leftover gas in the tank could be converted into oil, the human equivalent of fat.)

The second meaning of metabolism refers to the total amount of energy you spend in a given day. This, of course, changes as you age. If you're over 40, you know it takes more time to do things than when you were in your twenties. This is because you can't generate muscle power as fast as you used to.

Thus, the real culprit in having a difficult time maintaining your body weight is the reduction in metabolism only in this second sense of daily energy expenditure. Without a corresponding reduction in food intake, you may keep gaining weight. If you spend 100 fewer calories per day while consuming the same amount of calories as before, you can gain 10 pounds of weight a year. You could increase your calorie expenditure through exercise to try to prevent weight gain. However, you might not be able to sustain that level of activity.

10. What is the best way I can be sure of eating balanced meals?

Your body has a supply of nutrients in storage in addition to what is available in the blood. The body's internal sensors detect the need to replenish nutrients and inform the brain. When the brain decides it's the right time, you feel the sensation of hunger. No methodology currently available is able to determine the nutrient deficiencies in the body at any given time, even when you feel hungry. This means that, at present, there is no reliable way to eat exactly the right balanced diet to meet the body's current needs during each meal. Depending on the severity of deficiency and the concentration of nutrients in the food, it may take days of meals to restore your actual nutrient balance. This is why I suggest eating a variety of natural foods to ensure you have a better chance of ingesting the range of nutrients your body needs.

11. I don't like the mushy feeling in my mouth when I chew food thoroughly. What should I do to implement the idea of eating slowly and consciously?

When you're used to eating fast and swallowing food without chewing thoroughly, you may not actually know how a well-chewed piece of food feels in the mouth or how to savor the texture and qualities of the food you are eating. But by paying attention to your eating speed and noticing the feeling of food in your mouth as you start each meal, you will discover that you will begin to enjoy the food more, while also being more aware of how much you are consuming. Eating slowly and consciously, chewing every bite, also gives your brain a chance to register the nutrients in the food, helping to trigger the satisfaction signal telling you when to stop eating. Other satiation signals need more time to develop, such as signals from your stomach walls indicating they are full, and signals from your intestine and blood that tell the brain nutrients have arrived.

Paradoxically, when you chew slowly and realize that you don't like the mushy feeling, it is your brain telling you that you no longer need to eat because you have consumed enough. The sensation of no longer enjoying the food is, in fact, a signal to stop eating. If you are in doubt, take a few sips of water, clean your taste buds and decide whether you really feel like eating another bite.

If you constantly find yourself eating fast, it may mean that you have waited too long to eat. You need to ask yourself why you are skipping meals, and make adjustments so you can eat on a timely basis. If you notice that you are developing hunger at the end of a day when you have skipped lunch, snack on roasted nuts without salt as their digestion can moderate the intensity of your hunger.

If you find yourself absolutely famished, put a sugar-containing hard candy in your mouth and let it melt. This may reduce your hunger so that you won't reach home feeling starved, causing you to eat junk food or to gulp your meal down.

12. I have trouble following good eating habits when I'm at work, go to restaurants and dinner parties, or go on vacation. What can I do?

Changing your eating habits is a choice you must make, regardless of circumstances. Human nature is such that we are influenced by those around us. Co-workers wanting to share food with us, being in a restaurant surrounded by other people enjoying their enormous plates of food, having a friend invite us to dinner and offer up a sumptuous meal that he or she spent time making, lying on a beach at a tropical resort with all-you-can-eat meals—these are certainly all circumstances that can test your commitment to completely overhaul your eating habits to the extent recommended in Part 4 of this book.

But let me ask you this. When you drive a car, your goal is always safe driving, right? You would never say, "I have trouble driving safely when my co-workers are with me, when I drive to a restaurant, or when I go on vacation." So why would you change your commitment to healthier eating habits that maintain low blood sugar and prevent you from developing diabetes or reversing it in those other kinds of circumstances? Doesn't the quality of your own life provide the motivation you need to desire a life free from diabetes, rather than believing or feeling that you need to abandon your commitment because other people are around?

So when co-workers bring food to share at work and you feel that you don't want to disappoint the person, thank the person for their generosity and thoughtfulness, but let them know that you have medical reasons for not eating it, such as elevated blood sugar, high cholesterol, triglycerides, or a family history of diabetes. Hopefully, when they learn that you're serious about your health, they'll respect your decision and appreciate your sincerity. If they don't and insist that you eat the food with them, you might wonder why they are pressuring you and whether this is a good friend to listen to in matters related to food.

Similarly, when you are invited to at a dinner party, it is best to notify the host in advance of your food restrictions. If you are not able to do that and your host gives you a large plate of food, possibly with many carbohydrates you do not want to eat, you can certainly take a few bites to enjoy the offering. Do not feel obliged to eat everything on the plate. Again, let the host know about your commitment to better eating habits. In fact, find out if others at the table have high blood sugar or are concerned about diabetes. You might inspire an interesting discussion everyone will enjoy and learn from.

At restaurants, it can be easy to fall back into desiring your old favorite foods, and you may feel that you have to eat them given that you are paying for the meal. To counteract that, try to get in touch with your body's nutritional needs. What is your brain telling you to eat? Then eat slowly and consciously and try to leave 20 to 30 percent of the food on the plate. If you linger over the meal, your satisfaction signals will kick in about 20 to 30 minutes after the start of the meal and you'll discover that you are no longer hungry.

Finally, make your vacations times to rebuild your body's health, rather than put weight back on. Sample the variety of new foods you may encounter and remember to eat slowly and consciously because you have more time to savor the food. Avoid all-you-can eat resorts and cruises if you know these challenge your willpower and tempt you to overeat.

In the end, you have to take charge because no one other than you is responsible for your commitment to live a diabetes-free life.

A CALL TO ACTION

It is obvious that the lifestyles and diets of people throughout the world are promoting an increase, rather than a decrease, in the incidence of Type 2 diabetes, especially in the US. In fact, Dr. Leroy Hood, who helped pioneer the human genome project and is the president of the Institute for Systems Biology, stated at the January 23, 2015 meeting of the City Club of Portland that, based on a preliminary analysis of blood tests done every three months during the previous ten months, out of 100 adult volunteers who considered themselves healthy, 52 percent appeared headed to become diabetic. This is even higher than the American Diabetes Association statistics cited at the beginning of this book.

Scientists are conservative by nature and want to practice and build on what is already accepted in their field of expertise. Therefore, it is not surprising that experts who are proponents of the current concepts about diabetes are comfortable supporting the insulin resistance theory. However, a revolution occurs when a critical mass of people believing in a new ideology take action until the desired change is achieved. I would like to point out that I have come up with the new concepts in this book based on my own thinking and study, as yet to be verified through research. You must decide whether the theories and concepts make sense to you. If they do, then consider taking the following actions.

Talk to political leaders. Politicians too often act from an ideology and stick with it, sometimes for the benefit of their constituents, other times for their own benefit. For example, farmers want subsidies for growing grains and people want inexpensive foods to fit their budgets. Politicians vote subsidies through because they believe that farmers can help people have access to affordable grains and grain products. Unfortunately, they are agreeing to this without realizing they are helping fuel the spread of prediabetes and diabetes.

Decades ago, an experiment was done with Native Americans as the study subjects. They were transferred to reservations where, instead of their normal diet containing very little complex carbohydrate, they were asked to consume a majority of their energy intake in the form of grain products. Within a short period of time, relative to their long existence on this continent, they experienced the highest incidence of Type 2 diabetes of any other ethnic group in the US.

Today, through farm policies adopted by our government and supported by other parties with vested interests, this "experiment" is effectively being expanded to include all Americans and other populations around the globe who are also developing diabetes at an increasingly fast pace.

We must all begin telling politicians about this book and encouraging them to reconsider their support of grain subsidies by making use of the best scientific information currently available to decrease the incidence of Type 2 diabetes and related health care expenditures.

Change funding for research into diabetes. Government officials who allocate tax money for medical research should closely examine and even deny funding for any research involving the so-called insulin-resistance theory. This will clearly go against the wishes of the big pharmaceutical companies who want funding to support their theories because that explanation for high blood sugar and diabetes helps sell drugs. Instead, the government should begin supporting basic research to understand the mechanisms of bodily functions, including hunger, satiation, and the dispersal of nutrients in the body.

Review how doctors are taught. Sushruta, a 6th century BCE Indian healer, identified *Type 1* diabetes after noticing that ants were attracted to the urine of certain persons due to its sugar content. Later, elevated sugar level in the urine and blood found in patients with this condition were correlated with the absence of insulin production by the pancreas. This established Type 1 diabetes as a disease of the hormonal system.

When similar elevations of sugar were identified in the urine and blood of adults with Type 2 diabetes, it was natural to classify this as a hormonal disease, too. However, when it was found that the early stage of rising blood sugar in Type 2 diabetes was also associated with high levels of insulin circulating in the blood, it became necessary to produce an explanation. About 80 years ago, Dr William Falta proposed the theory of "insulin resistance" as one possible explanation. Immediate acceptance of this theory by the endocrinologists solidified the classification of Type 2 diabetes as an endocrine disease. But is it?

Science thrives on challenging even entrenched concepts and advances with each change based on solid evidence. We accept one theory about how something happens until evidence suggests that this theory is wrong, and another must take its place. I believe we are at this juncture when it comes to continuing to accept that insulin resistance is the cause of Type 2 diabetes. Editors of medical textbooks should show courage and classify Type 2 diabetes as a form of nutrition overload rather than as an endocrine disease.

Change how doctors treat diabetes. We must ask medical professionals who prescribe insulin to treat Type 2 diabetes because of the "progressive nature of this illness" to show proof that insulin shots halt the progression. Medical treatment of Type 2 diabetes should be based on beneficial outcomes for the patient, such as a reduced incidence of problems related to the heart, eye, kidney and other organs, rather than on the evidence that the treatment reduces blood sugar values.

Move away from treating diabetes with drugs. The primary objective of prediabetes therapy should transition away from drugs to teaching people to empty out their fat cells so that excess glucose could be transferred into them after conversion to triglyceride by the liver. The secondary objective should be to reduce accumulation of fat in the blood circulation to prevent blockage of blood vessels that can result in damage to the heart and brain. The third objective should be to protect the integrity of tiny blood vessels in the eye, kidneys, and feet so that they do not suffer damage. Any medication that can produce hypoglycemia, induce the sensation of hunger, increase blood fat, or lead to significant weight gain should be avoided or used only on a short-term basis.

Update recommendations about body weight standards. We must challenge the medical community to reassess the basis and reasoning underlying the current recommendations for ideal body weight and the averages recommended for the intake of the food groups. Both of these measures are misleading and generally miss the point of healthy eating.

Stop confusing the public about grains. We need to question those who advocate consumption of "whole grains" over "refined grains," as this actually provides no benefit for consumers. *Grains, no matter how whole they are, still result in glucose in the bloodstream.*

Raise awareness among nutritional specialists. We need specialists in nutrition, not specialists who practice medicine for a living, to begin setting dietary guidelines based on acquisition of nutrients by the body rather than based on food groups.

Educate the public. We must ask professionals who initially interact with people in a health care setting, such as nurse practitioners, family doctors, pediatricians, internists, obstetricians and other providers to begin giving individualized instructions to each and every American on nutrition and the acquisition of nutrients—and then follow up with their patients in subsequent visits.

Teach families how to truly "enjoy" food. We need to educate families about their food choices when shopping and cooking. When shopping for fruits and vegetables, don't buy based only on their appearance; look for information on their nutrient content or get a sample to assess their flavor. Cooking should be actively promoted as a shared family activity, starting with the adventure of finding fresh, natural ingredients containing a full complement of nutrients as nature intended and using foods and exotic spices based on recipes from different regions of the world where food is more healthy and natural than in the US.

Take responsibility for yourself. Become educated about your own responsibility for the food you eat and serve, realizing that your choices lead to disease when you overeat consistently, and especially when you consume too much grain-based carbohydrates, salt, and sugar. I invite you to read and sign the pledge at the end of this book, certifying that you are making a pact with yourself to live longer and keep diabetes out of your life.

This book has emphasized the fact that everyone is born with an internal regulatory system to regulate the intake of nutrients for a lifetime, starting with the selection of food items based on intuition rather than on the recommendations of experts. This is because only your brain is knowledgeable regarding the nutrient status of *your* body. You must listen when your brain generates the sensation of hunger because this is the alarm indicating that the combined deficiencies of different nutrients have reached a threshold level. This is when you should eat, and only then. Your hunger will vary day by day because the type and degree of deficiencies change from one hunger sensation to another.

This book also advocates cultivating your awareness of nutrient overload. Overconsumption is directly linked to high blood sugar and the risks of getting diabetes. The keys to weight maintenance and preventing diabetes have to do with consuming a variety of nutrients and creating enjoyment in the process of eating, ultimately leading to the feeling of satisfaction. You must deemphasize the consumption of grain and grain-based products by not making or serving them.

Research shows that people who reduce their body weight by just 5 to 7 percent can significantly improve their odds of not developing Type 2 diabetes after they are diagnosed with prediabetes. Eliminating the risks of diabetes in Americans can no longer be based on the conventional paradigm of balancing energy input with energy output, such as through exercise, or using an external control of your energy-containing food consumption to achieve weight maintenance, such as through some company's diet program. Neither of these solutions has been shown to be effective in the long-term for the majority of people with high blood sugar and/or who are overweight.

Since we cannot define what a healthy person should look like, we have to be nonjudgmental of people's appearances. This will take time, so we need to muster forces to begin immediate change. Through the media, government agencies, parenting groups, and our schools and universities, our collective emphasis must turn to teaching children to be conscious of their own bodies and to educate them about the existence of different body shapes and appearances. In addition, parents need support to accept their children's physical appearance, as long as they are healthy. Adults should set an example and respect the physical appearance of their peers.

It will take a revolutionary change in what we eat and how we eat, with each of us contributing our share to limit the production, distribution, and consumption of grain products, to stop the progression of diabetes in our lifetime. Each of us goes through multiple life stages, beginning with infancy and ending with the winding down of our life. In this book, I am offering you the chance to avoid living out your life as a diabetic.

Your feeling of empowerment should start with the realization that the human body is designed to tolerate deprivation better than to survive an overload of nutrients, especially carbohydrates, by virtue of its ability to use fatty acids as fuel and convert amino acids into glucose. The next step is to exercise the right to enjoy what you eat with the confidence that your brain knows what your nutrient needs are and will inform you when you have had enough. The more you feel your chewing motions, the more you will fulfill the objective of a meal: *enjoying more of what you eat*. The success of a meal should not be based on how much you eat, but how much you enjoy what you eat.

Understand the nature of products made from whole grains as sugar molecules with additional nutrients, nutrients easily available from other natural sources. Don't be persuaded by secondary advertising claims such as "no cholesterol," "gluten free," "fortified with vitamins and minerals," and "no high-fructose corn syrup" because such claims do not change the basic composition of these products; they are still foods that will elevate your blood sugar. As you learn, teach the people around you how they can become part of the revolution to change the way we live, eat and enjoy.

THE EAT, CHEW, LIVE PLEDGE

The best way to reduce your risk of diabetes is to reflect on this book and recognize the impact that it can have on your life. If you have understood the science explained in this book, agree with the reasoning presented, and feel motivated to start the program, you need to commit to a plan to sustain your motivation. I invite you to write the following pledge with your own hand on two pieces of paper, one small enough to be carried in your wallet and the other large enough to be displayed on your refrigerator or pantry door to remind yourself of your commitment to a diabetes-free life.

THE EAT, CHEW, LIVE
DIABETES-FREE PLEDGE

The conscious mind of

_____
(your name here)

does hereby pledge to the physical body of

_____
(your name here)

to protect you from the ravages of Type 2 diabetes,

(a privilege currently denied to many),

until the end of our natural life together.

■

I will not only help you to age gracefully,

free from the risk of a life cut short by diabetes-related

complications, but also help you experience the

true enjoyment and pleasure of eating.

Dr. Poothullil's analysis and perspective of Type 2 diabetes is refreshingly courageous, and questions the conformist wisdom of what typical doctors tell their patients. More importantly, as a diabetic and a layperson, I found Dr. Poothullil's advice on seriously eliminating carbohydrates, mindful eating, and chewing to be effective and feasible routines to adopt.

Satya, Type 2 Diabetic, Oregon

GLOSSARY

Acetyl coenzyme A An important molecule that is essential to the balance between carbohydrate metabolism and fat metabolism. The acetyl coenzyme A released from fatty acids inside muscle cells provides fuel for the production of energy.

Active muscle cells Cells that have become warm or activated through exercise. Active muscle cells can immediately absorb glucose without help from insulin.

Adenosine triphosphate (ATP) A molecule found in all cells. All living things require energy to function, but the energy must be transformed into a form the body can easily use. ATP acts as a chemical battery that stores energy. This energy is released when needed.

Adrenaline A hormone released from the adrenal glands during stress, excitement or fasting. Adrenaline facilitates the conversion of triglycerides to fatty acids for use by the muscles.

Amino acids Organic compounds that are absorbed after the digestion of proteins in the intestine. The liver converts amino acids that are not immediately used into glucose.

Amylase An enzyme that digests starch into sugar. It is secreted by the salivary glands and the pancreas.

Atherosclerosis Buildup of plaque in and on the walls of the arteries, reducing blood flow. The plaque is composed of fats, cholesterol, and other substances.

Authentic weight The body weight at which your brain knows it is operating at optimal health.

Bile salts A thick fluid synthesized by the liver from cholesterol and secreted by the gallbladder. Bile salts promote the absorption of fats in the intestine.

Biological mechanisms A system by which a living organism changes itself.

Blood sugar The amount of sugar in your blood. Carbohydrates from food break down into glucose, a form of sugar. When glucose is absorbed, your blood sugar level climbs.

Brown fat One of the two types of fat in the body. Newborns have far more brown fat than adults. Brown fat cells generate heat, rather than just store fat as in other fat cells.

Carbohydrate-based fat replacers Substances used by food manufacturers to replace the taste and function of fats in food, but containing fewer calories.

Carbohydrates A large group of organic compounds found in bread, noodles, potatoes, and fruit. Carbohydrates break down into sugar or glucose in the body.

Carnitine A substance found in every cell in the body. Carnitine escorts fatty acids into the mitochondria that break them to release ATP.

Cells All of the organs and tissue in our body are composed of cells, the smallest and most basic structural and biological unit of life. Cells take in nutrients, convert nutrients into energy, and carry out specialized functions.

Cholesterol A waxy substance that is produced by the body, and also comes from food. The cholesterol from food is a nutrient consisting of a molecule of fat.

Complex carbohydrates Carbohydrates consisting of more than two sugar molecules, created by a bond between carbon atom number 1 of one glucose molecule and carbon atom number 4 of another glucose molecule.

Cortisol A hormone released from the adrenal gland. Cortisol stimulates fat cells to release fatty acids from fat. It enhances the burning of fatty acids, and stimulates the liver to produce glucose from amino acids.

Dehydration A condition that occurs when the body loses more fluid than it takes in.

Diabetic coma In type 2 diabetes, this type of coma occurs due to very high blood sugar that results in a loss of body fluid and dehydration.

Dopamine A chemical released by the brain that transmits signals between the brain's nerve cells, causing a pleasurable feeling.

Endocrine function of the pancreas The secretion of two main hormones the body needs to regulate blood sugar: insulin and glucogen.

Exocrine function of the pancreas The secretion of digestive hormones in the small intestine by the pancreas that help break down carbohydrates, proteins and fats in food.

Fat A nutrient found in foods such as oil, butter and meats. Fat breaks down into fatty acids in the body.

Fat cells Cells in your body that store excess triglycerides (fat).

Fatty acid burn theory Alternative theory for cause of Type 2 diabetes, presented in this book.

Fatty acids If glucose is not available, most cells in the body can use fatty acids as fuel to produce energy.

Gestational diabetes The sudden development of diabetes during pregnancy.

Glucagon A hormone from the pancreas that prompts the liver to release glucose.

Glucose A form of sugar. Primary fuel for muscles, brain cells, and red blood cells.

Glycation Attachment of glucose molecules to different proteins in the body. Too much glycation causes impairment of cell function.

Glycerol A molecule needed to produce fat called triglyceride from the fatty acids.

Glycogen An insoluble storage form of glucose produced in the liver that can be broken back down to glucose when the body needs it.

Grain-based carbohydrates Includes all the complex starch foods of the grain family - wheat, oats, barley, corn, rice, and rye.

Grehlin A hormone released by cells in the stomach that increases the intensity of hunger.

Growth hormone A hormone produced in the pituitary gland that helps children grow. In adults, growth hormone is released when exercising or under stress.

High blood sugar A medical term for too much glucose in the blood.

High-density lipoprotein (HDL) Lipoproteins are special particles composed of proteins that attach to fat (lipids). The liver can change the high-density lipo-proteins associated with a cholesterol molecule to low-density lipoproteins and vise versa.

High-fructose corn syrup A liquid sweetener added to many foods and beverages as an alternative to sugar. It enhances the taste and increases the palatability, presentation, aroma, and texture of food.

Hormone A type of chemical that is made in one part of the body, but is carried to other parts of the body through the blood to produce a desired effect.

Hyperglycemia A condition in which there is too much glucose in the blood.

Hypoglycemia A condition in which there is too little glucose in the blood.

Inactive muscle cells Muscles that have rested and are cooled down. Cool muscles cannot absorb glucose without the help of insulin.

Insulin A hormone produced in the pancreas that enables glucose to move from the bloodstream into cells.

Insulin resistance theory The current medical theory for the cause of Type 2 diabetes, proposing that the cells become resistant to insulin's message.

Insulin sensitivity The response of cells to the presence of insulin.

Lactose One of the three natural forms of sugar, lactose is composed of one molecule each of glucose and galactose. It is found in milk and milk products.

Lipase An enzyme that helps break down fats in food into fatty acids.

Low-density lipoprotein (LDL) Protein articles, which are produced in the liver and attached to fat. When there is excess LDL cholesterol in the body, it can adhere to the lining of arteries, causing the buildup of plaque.

Macronutrients Nutrients needed by the body in large amounts. The main macronutrients are proteins, fats, and carbohydrates.

Maltose One of the three natural sugars in food, maltose is a double sugar unit containing two glucose molecules.

Metabolism Metabolism is the chemical reactions of energy and matter in the body needed to maintain life.

Micronutrients Nutrients that the body needs in very small amounts.

Mindful eating Eating slowly and with awareness of the taste and texture of the food.

Mitochondria Mitochondria convert food into energy, called ATP, for the cell to use. Mitochondria are found in nearly all cells. Numerous mitochondria are found in very active cells such as a liver cell.

Monounsaturated fats A type of dietary, unsaturated fat, found in foods such as olive oil and nuts.

Muscle cells The muscles in your body are composed of muscle cells.

No-calorie sweeteners They are stevia, aspartame, sucralose, neotame, acesulfame potassium (Ace-K), saccharin, advantame and cyclamates.

Pancreas A glandular organ composed of exocrine cells that excrete digestive enzymes, and endocrine cells that excrete hormones such as insulin and glucagon.

Polyunsaturated fats A type of unsaturated, dietary fat. The fat molecules have more than one unsaturated carbon bond in the molecule. Common sources of this type of fat are salmon, walnuts, flax, sunflower oil, sesame seeds, and olive oil.

Prediabetes A blood sugar level that is between 5.7 and 6.4% on a test called the A1C. The A1C level of a full diabetic is over 6.5%.

Proteins Nutrients found in foods and break down into amino acids in body.

Red blood cells Blood cells that carry oxygen throughout the body.

Saturated fats A type of dietary fat that is called saturated because of its chemical structure. It is usually a solid at room temperature. Lard, butter, coconut oil, palm oil, palm kernel oil, whole milk, red meat and full-fat cheese all contain saturated fats.

Skeletal muscles Muscles that connect to the skeleton. Skeletal muscle consumes 80 to 90 percent of the glucose from food.

Sodium One of the chemical components in salt. The other component is chloride. The body cannot absorb complex carbohydrates without sodium.

Starch A form of complex carbohydrate composed of long strings of glucose with branches that also have long strings of glucose

Statin medicines A class of medicines used to lower cholesterol.

Stem cells Cells in the body that can turn into other types of cells when needed, such as fat cells.

Sucrose One of the three natural forms of sugar, composed of one glucose molecule and one fructose molecule. It is found in fruits, berries, sugar cane, and sugar beets.

Treatment modalities In medicine, treatment modalities refers to the methods by which diseases are treated.

Triglycerides Fat produced by combining three fatty acids to a molecule of glycerol.

Type 1 diabetes Also called juvenile-onset diabetes. An illness in which the pancreatic cells that produce insulin have been destroyed by immune cells, and the body is unable to produce enough insulin as a result.

Type 2 diabetes The most common form of diabetes, in which the pancreas still produces insulin, but there is a buildup of glucose in the blood. Often called adult-onset diabetes.

Unsaturated fats A fat or fatty acid in which there is one or more than one double bond in the fatty acid chain.

Whole grain products Products made with grains containing the bran, germ, and endosperm of the plant.

ACKNOWLEDGMENTS

I would like to thank Irma, Tammy and Rhonda for assisting with research. I also thank Dr. Venugopal Menon, Dr. Antony Poothullil, Dr. Ramanathan, Dr. Kay Bauman, Dr. Stephen LaFranchi, Dr. A.E. Daniel, Dr. Gerry Brown, Janet Meirelles, Mr. Jacob Mundaden, and George Kannarkat for their comments, reviews, and helpful suggestions on the manuscript.

I also want to thank my publishers at Over And Above Creative Group, especially Rick Benzel for his insight and guidance in developing this book, and Susan Shankin for her beautiful design work and Tanya Maiboroda for the interior design. For the illustrations in this book, I extend my gratitude to Tim Kummerow for the wonderful cover illustration and storyboard art inserts, and Cristian Voicu for the spot art drawings. I also thank Marian Pierce for her many reviews and careful copyediting of the manuscript. Finally, I thank Julia and Jared Drake at Julia Drake Public Relations for their work helping me promote the important message of this book.

About the Author

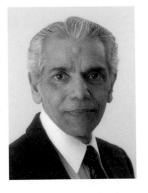

John M. Poothullil, MD, FRCP practiced medicine as a pediatrician and allergist for more than 30 years, with 27 of those years in the state of Texas. He received his medical degree from the University of Kerala, India in 1968, after which he did two years of medical residency in Washington, DC and Phoenix, AZ and two years of fellowship, one in Milwaukee, Wisconsin and the other in Ontario, Canada. He began his practice in 1974 and retired in 2008. He holds certifications from the American Board of Pediatrics, The American Board of Allergy & Immunology, and the Canadian Board of Pediatrics.

During his medical practice, John became interested in understanding the causes of and interconnections between hunger, satiation, and weight gain. His interest turned into a passion and a multi-decade personal study and research project that led him to read many medical journal articles, medical textbooks, and other scholarly works in biology, biochemistry, physiology, endocrinology, and cellular metabolic functions. This eventually guided Dr. Poothullil to investigate the theory of insulin resistance as it relates to diabetes. Recognizing that this theory was illogical, he spent several years rethinking the biology behind high blood sugar and developed the fatty acid burn theory as the real cause of diabetes.

Dr. Poothullil has written articles on hunger and satiation, weight loss, diabetes, and the senses of taste and smell. His articles have been published in medical journals such as *Physiology and Behavior, Neuroscience and Biobehavioral Reviews, Journal of Women's Health, Journal of Applied Research, Nutrition,* and *Nutritional Neuroscience.* His work has been quoted in *Woman's Day, Fitness, Red Book* and *Woman's World.*

■

Please visit www.eatchewlive.com to follow Dr. Poothullil's blog and to send us your questions and feedback on how *Eat, Chew, Live* has changed your life.